BIG GREEN EGG

CERAMIC CHARCOAL GRILL

COOKBOOK 1000

THE COMPLETE GUIDE TO 1000 DAYS TRIED & TRUE RECIPES

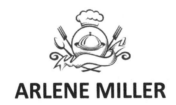

ARLENE MILLER

CONTENTS

INTRODUCTION..8

How Does A Kamado Grill Work? 8

The Benefits of the Big Green Egg Kamado Grill 8

How to Use Your Big Green Egg Kamado Grill.......................10

How to Deeply Clean Your Big Green Egg Kamado Grill 12

FISH AND SEAFOOD 13

Seared Ahi Tuna 13

Morro Bay Bbq Cowboy Oysters 13

Scallops With Pea-sto 14

Grilled Asian Mahi-mahi 14

Smoked King Salmon 15

Grilled Fish Tacos With Peach Salsa 16

Cedar-plank Salmon..17

Marinated Grilled Salmon..18

Lemon Bed Cod 18

Black Pepper Dungeness Crab 19

Grilled Tuna With Herb Butter..20

Fish And Shrimp Stuffed Jalapeños 21

Scallops, Asparagus And Artichoke Gratin...............................22

Grilled Shrimp And Taylor Farms Tangerine Crunch Wraps 22

Bacon-wrapped Cod With Roasted Potatoes And Baby Arugula Salad.......23

Red Fish Pot Pie..24

Florida Lobster Roll 25

Grilled Lobster Tails 25

Hatch Chili Shrimp And Grits 26

Cedar-planked Salmon..27

Greek Sea Bass 27

Grilled Caribbean Snapper With Vera Cruz Salsa 28

Herb Butter Lobster Tails..29

Ginger Scallion Scallops...29

Country Ham, Shrimp & Grits Kabobs 30

POULTRY 31

Grill Glazed Sweet Asian Chicken Pan Grill 31

Brined Roasted Turkey 32

Grilled Hot Candy Chicken Wings 33

Grilled Pheasant With Chimichurri 33

Bbq Chicken Cheddar Sandwich 34

Green Tomato Pizza With Smoked Chicken And Truffle Crema.........................35

Chicken Cacciatore 37

Jerk Chicken Wings 37

Wild Rice Turkey Biryani Stuffed Whole Pumpkin 38

Wasabi Honey Teriyaki Grilled Chicken Thighs..40

Greg Bates Bbq Chicken 40

Vidalia Onion And Sriracha-glazed Nashville Hot Wings................................41

Rathbun Chicken 41

Butter-injected Turkey And Sides 42

Green Curry Chicken 43

Smokey Thai Pulled Chicken Sandwiches 44

Bbq Chicken Soup..46

Jamaican Jerk Chicken Wings 47

Ultimate Chicken Curry 48

Grilled Chicken Arugula Pesto Wings 49

Greek Isles Marinated Chicken...50

Beer Can Chicken 51

Smoky Grilled Chicken Wings 52

Cuban Chicken Bombs 53

Walk The Plank Chicken Quarters 53

BEEF **54**

Surf And Turf Rolls 54

Smoked Beef Tenderloin..55

Italian Meatballs..56

Smoked Canuck Chili 57

Moroccan Meatball Sliders...58

Smoked Beef Brisket 59

Corned Beef And Cabbage..59

Smash Cheese Burgers 60

Frankie Ballard's Rib-eye Steaks...60

Homemade Pastrami 61

Smoked Brisket Roll..62

Grilled Italian Meatloaf Sandwich 63

Dr. Bbq's Roasted Upside Down Chili 64

Taco Soup 65

Italian Sausage Sliders 65

Grilled Top Blade Steak 66

The Perfect Steak 67

Pitmaster Ribeyes 67

Ancho Chili Steak Tacos 68

Braised Short Ribs 68

Bacon-wrapped Steakhouse Filet 69

Reverse Sear Tri Tip With Chimichurri 69

Pulled Beef Sandwich 70

Rouladen 71

BURGERS 72

Breakfast Burger 72

Classic American Burger 73

Oahu Burger 73

Quesadilla Burger 74

The Crowned Jewels Burger 75

"the Masterpiece" 76

DESSERTS 77

Grilled Fruit Pie 77

Berry Upside-down Cake 78

Corn & Jalapeño Focaccia 79

Seasonal Fruit Cobbler 80

Chocolate Chip Cookie Peanut Butter Cup S'mores 80

Fresh Peach Crisp 81

Brownies 81

Pizza Margherita 82

Caramel Cinnamon Rolls 83

Grilled Sopapillas 83

Whole Apples With Caramel Sauce 84

Almond Cream Cake 85

Peaches And Pound Cake 86

3 Ingredient Fruit Cobbler 86

Grilled Plums With Honey And Ricotta 87

Grilled Naan 87

Upside Down Triple Berry Pie 88

Death By Chocolate 88

Sourdough Baguette 89

Lemon Poppy Seed Cake 90

Best Banana Bread..91

Peach Dutch Baby..91

Apple Cake..92

Peanut Butter Bacon Bars..92

SIDES **93**

Soba Noodle Bowl..93

Prosciutto And Pear Bruschetta 94

Broiled Tomatoes And Parmesan..94

Lasagna...95

Roasted Potatoes 95

Mac And Cheese..96

Summer Squash & Eggplant..97

Parmesan Zucchini Spears...97

Smoked Potato Salad...98

Sweet Potato Fries...98

Sweet Potato Bake..99

Breakfast Casserole...99

Corn & Poblano Pudding..100

Cowboy Caviar...100

Baba Ganoush 101

Campfire Potato Salad 102

Bacon Wrapped Pineapple 102

Grilled Vegetable Succotash...103

Grilled Artichokes..104

Arroz A La Mexicana (mexican Rice)...105

Mojito Watermelon..105

Grilled Sweet Potatoes...106

German Potato Salad 106

Grilled Watermelon Salad..107

Thanksgiving Stuffing..107

PORK...**108**

Pork Tenderloin 108

Pork Belly & Rice Grits 109

Pork Chops..110

Pork Cacciatore 112

Cedar Planked Pork Chops 113

Potato Salad With Bacon 114

Bacon-wrapped Scotch Eggs...115

Bacon Mac & Cheese 116

Maple Bourbon Pork Chops 117

Baby Back Ribs With Apple-bourbon Barbecue Sauce 118

Reverse-seared Herb Crusted Bone-in Iberico Pork Loin 120

Citrus Pork Loin 121

Dr. Bbq's Pork Chops 122

Smoked Spareribs 123

Pork T-bone With Walnut Bulgur Pilaf 124

Cedar Plank Pork Tenderloin 125

Smoked Ham On Grill 125

Ham Muffinini 126

Cuban Pork (lechon Asado) 126

Christmas Gingersnap Ham 127

Virginia Willis Pulled Pork 128

INTRODUCTION

How Does A Kamado Grill Work?

A kamado is no ordinary barbecue. Its strength lies partly in the combination of the oval shape and the possibility to regulate the air flow. Ceramic kamados also have the advantage of the material, which insulates and reflects heat.

You need to close the lid during cooking. This has to be done after each action and with every cooking technique. As soon as the lid is closed, the shape of the kamado creates a current of hot air. Because only some of the air can escape, the heat circulates around the ingredient or dish, a bit like a charcoal-fired convection oven. By closing the lid, you make sure that as little heat as possible is lost and that the ceramic barbecue maintains the desired temperature. This gives you good control over the cooking process.

The Benefits of the Big Green Egg Kamado Grill

There are several ways Kamado Grills can benefit the backyard griller who is looking to enhance their outdoor cooking experience:

1. Versatility

Kamado Grills are exceptional for grilling, smoking, baking, BBQ, and roasting. This versatility allows the outdoor cook many unique options in one grill.

Feel like making a true wood fired pizza ? Because of its design, kamado grills make exceptional pizza ovens since they are extremely efficient at insulating and circulating heat throughout the grill. This results in a crispy bottom crust while perfectly melting the top layer of cheese.

And don't forget about the classics either. Steaks, ribs, burgers, the Kamado can cook them all with that classic lump charcoal flavor.

2. Flavor

Kamado Grills use wood lump charcoal which results in a tasty smoke and charcoal flavor that is classically associated with grilling.

Ceramic charcoal grills also do a tremendous job at retaining the moisture of whatever you are cooking. Since air is locked tightly, your meat remains more tender and juicier than it would on a regular charcoal grill.

3. Steady Temperatures

Since Kamado Grills are so well insulated, temperatures hold relatively steady for longer periods of time compared to a traditional charcoal grill. There is a learning curve to controlling temperatures as you will need to play around with the dampers to balance the intake and outflow of air.

In short: More air = more heat, less air = less heat.

4. Longevity

As champion Pit Master Chris Lilly states quite perfectly

"Ask your children what color they want, because they will inherit it."

As long as you treat your Kamado with care (and don't drop it from a height where it can crack), it should last a very long time.

5. Maintenance is Simple

Cleaning and maintaining a Kamado Grill is a breeze. Simply clean your grates and gently brush out the bottom. The ceramic is self-cleaning so do not use a wire brush as they can damage the surface.

6. A Great Grill for the Winter

Because Kamados are constructed to have such effective insulation, cold temperatures do not have the same effect on internal temperatures as it does on other grills. You may have to use more fuel to bring your grill up to its desired temperature, but once it reaches that temp, it will hold much better than a standard charcoal or propane grill.

How to Use Your Big Green Egg Kamado Grill

1. Looftlighter or Electric Starter

Perhaps the easiest way to light your charcoal is with a powered heat source.

Electric starters have been around for decades, and they're simple to operate. Using an electric heating element not unlike what you'll find on a stovetop to ignite the coals, you just plug it in, turn it on, and wait.

A Looftlighter is, essentially, the world's most intense blow dryer. It employs super-heated air and a powerful fan to heat charcoal until it fires up. Not going to lie – they're pretty cool.

2. Pyramid Method

This is a classic strategy used in standard charcoal grills. All you have to do is pile your charcoal in a pyramid shape and insert two or three fire starters. Just light the fire starters, and soon they will fire up the charcoal.

With a regular grill, you'd want to spread your charcoal around, but since we want a pyramid shape anyway, there's no need to touch anything after lighting.

3. Chimney Starter

If you have a traditional charcoal grill, there's a pretty good chance you already own a chimney starter. If you don't here's a quick synopsis of how they work:

A chimney starter is a cylinder of metal with a handle on one side, and a grate about three-quarters of the way down on the inside. You fill the large side of the cylinder with charcoal and stuff the small, bottom section with newspaper and set the whole thing down on a fireproof surface.

Light up the paper, and before long, the charcoal will catch. Once it's nicely smoldering, carefully pour the coals into your firebox and arrange.

Of the three methods, we most recommend using a Looftlighter or fire starters. While chimneys are great, it can be awkward to pour the lit coals into your Kamado and then arrange them properly.

4. A Word on Lighting Fluids

If you and charcoal grilling go way back, there's a good chance you've used lighting fluids. Time was, it was pretty much standard practice for cookouts.

Simply squirt a flammable liquid on your briquettes, and light it up. As the fluid burned off, it set the briquettes to smoldering.

Yes, it works like a charm. It's also a bit dangerous if you're not careful.

The biggest problem, however, is it can add a nasty chemical taste to your food. You didn't just shell out big bucks for a kamado to eat brisket with an aftertaste of kerosene, now did you?

In a standard grill, you can get away with using an accelerant, then letting the coals rip until every single one is burning and ashed over. At this point, you can be sure all accelerant has burned away.

With many cooking techniques in a kamado, however, you only have a small portion of charcoal lit, and close down the vents to keep a lower temperature. The fire then spreads coal to coal over many hours, allowing a very long, low n slow cook.

This means, however, that any accelerant used will not have burned off and will be present to taint the flavor of your food.

So our recommendation: **NEVER** use lighting fluids in a Kamado cooker.

5. Flip Your Lid and Open Your Vents

As we've said, you need oxygen for the fire to burn. Controlling the flow of air into and out of your Kamado is the key to adjusting the temperature.

For now, though, open the bottom vent all the way and leave the lid open to get your charcoal burning.

After about 10 minutes, close the lid, but fully open the top vent. In general, you should start closing your vents when you're about 50F (28C) below your target, but we'll have more specific instructions on this later.

How to Deeply Clean Your Big Green Egg Kamado Grill

So the time has come to get stuck into a deep clean on your kamado grill.

For all the regular ash removal and mold cleaning you do, it's still important to do a deep clean on your kamado every few months.

Don't worry though. This is a lot more straightforward than you might think, and can easily be broken down into just a few steps.

1. Place all components such as cooking grates and deflector plates in their allotted place in the grill.
2. Heat up the grill with the lid closed and air vents/dampers wide open. Aim for about 500-600°F.
3. Allow the grill to stay at this temperature for about 30 minutes, before then closing the vents and allow the grill to cool down.
4. Once the grill has cooled, open the lid and remove the grill grates and deflector plates. The long exposure to the heat will have burned away much of the dirt and grease, but you will then have to use a grill brush to clean away the rest. Don't use any soap, water or chemicals for this.
5. Remove any coal inside the kamado, and then take out any other components in the grill.
6. Remove any residual ash. This can most efficiently be done with a vacuum clean. Follow this up by using a slightly damp cloth or paper towel to pick up any stubborn ash.
7. Remove the ash tray and empty it.
8. Put all components back in the grill, and place lid back on grill.

And that's it. It's a lot easier than people think, and only needs to be done once or twice a year. In comparison to regular charcoal or gas grills, kamado grills are far easier to clean and lower maintenance.

FISH AND SEAFOOD

Seared Ahi Tuna

Servings:2
Cooking Time: 6 Minutes

Ingredients:

- 2 ahi tuna steaks
- ¼ cup soy sauce
- 1 teaspoon corn starch
- ¼ cup pineapple juice
-
- ¼ cup honey
- 1 teaspoon sriracha
- 2 tablespoons sesame seeds, toasted

Directions:

1. Preheat the grill to 500°F using direct heat with a cast iron grate installed. Mix soy sauce and cornstarch until smooth. Add pineapple juice, honey and sriracha. Place pot on stove over medium heat and bring to a boil. Reduce heat and simmer 3-4 minutes until the thickened. Remove from heat.
2. Heat cast iron skillet and add oil. Sear tuna steaks 1-2 minutes, brushing each side with sauce mixture after searing. Garnish with sesame seeds.

Morro Bay Bbq Cowboy Oysters

Servings:6
Cooking Time: 10 Minutes

Ingredients:

- 6 Morro Bay Jumbo Oysters, washed well
- ¼ lb butter
- 1 large shallot
- A "good splash" of bourbon
- 2 teaspoons your favorite BBQ spice
- Lemon
- ½ bunch chives, sliced

Directions:

1. Preheat the grill to 400°F using direct heat with a cast iron grate installed. In a small saucepot, sauté shallots in a bit of butter. Add BBQ spice and then flambé with bourbon. Add a squeeze of lemon and then reserve sauce for when the oysters open. Place oysters on grill with the cup of the oyster flame side down. Put lid down and cook until they just pop open, about 5 minutes. When oysters open and they will stick to the top shell, shuck then into your bourbon pan sauce. Add a little of the oyster liqueur as well. Take a pair of kitchen scissors and cut the oysters in half or into bite size pieces. Place oysters back into the bottom shell and when ready re-fire on the grill Garnish with sliced chives, a pinch of BBQ spice and a little something crispy!

Scallops With Pea-sto

Servings: 4

Cooking Time: 7 Minutes

Ingredients:

- 1-lb sea scallops
- 2 Tablespoons olive oil
- Salt and Pepper
- Pea-sto
- 1 cup fresh green peas, blanched (you can also use frozen peas that have been thawed)
- 1/2 cup pecorino romano cheese, grated
- 1/4 cup basil leaves
- 1/4 cup mint leaves
- 3/4 tsp salt
- 1/2 tsp pepper
- 1/4 tsp crushed red chile flakes
- Olive oil

Directions:

1. In a food processor, combine peas, basil, mint, salt, pepper, and chile flakes and process until smooth. Add cheese.
2. Add enough olive oil until the pea-sto becomes a sauce-like consistency (about 1/2 cup). Set aside.
3. Grilling:
4. Preheat the grill to 400°F using direct heat with a cast iron grate installed.
5. Brush both sides of the scallops with olive oil and season with salt and pepper.
6. Place scallops on the grill and closer the dome for 3 minutes.
7. Gently flip the scallops and lower the dome for an additional 2-4 minutes.
8. Remove the scallops and pour some of the pea-sto on top.
9. Additional pea-sto can be saved in the fridge for 3 days. (It's delicious on pasta!)

Grilled Asian Mahi-mahi

Servings:4

Cooking Time: 24 Minutes

Ingredients:

- 4 (1 inch thick) Mahi-Mahi filets
- 1 tablespoon Better Than Bouillon Fish Base
- 1/2 cup soy sauce
- 1 1/2 Tablespoon sesame oil
- 1 teaspoon honey
- 1/2 teaspoon garlic powder
- 2 teaspoons sesame seeds

Directions:

1. Preheat the grill to 400°F using direct heat with a cast iron grate installed.
2. Mix the fish base, soy sauce, sesame oil, honey and garlic powder in a medium-sized shallow bowl. Add the Mahi-Mahi to the bowl and marinate for 20 minutes.
3. Place the Mahi-Mahi directly onto the kamado grill and grill for 3-4 minutes per side.
4. Remove the fish from the grill, sprinkle with the sesame seeds and serve immediately.

Smoked King Salmon

Servings: 8

Cooking Time: 75 Minutes

Ingredients:

- 2lb (1kg) skinless King salmon fillets
- for the brine
- 1/2 cup kosher salt
- 1/2 cup packed light brown sugar
- 3 tbsp pickling spice
- 6 cups hot water
- for the pesto
- 5 tbsp extra virgin olive oil, divided
- 1/4 cup walnut halves
- 2 cups baby arugula, loosely packed
- 1 cup fresh basil leaves, loosely packed
- 3 tbsp freshly grated Parmigiano-Reggiano
- 1 garlic clove
- kosher salt and freshly ground black pepper
- to smoke
- alder or cedar wood chunks

Directions:

1. To make the brine, in a medium bowl, whisk together salt, brown sugar, pickling spice, and water until salt and sugar have dissolved. Add ice cubes until the liquid is no longer hot. Place salmon in a resealable plastic bag, add the brine to cover, and refrigerate for 30 minutes. (Any extra brine can be refrigerated and saved for a later use.)

2. Remove salmon from the brine, pat dry with paper towels, and refrigerate until the surface begins to look dry and feel slightly tacky, about 30 to 60 minutes more.

3. Preheat the grill to 225°F (107°C) using indirect heat. Once hot, add the wood chunks and install a cast iron grate and a cast iron skillet. Place 1 tbsp oil and walnuts in the skillet, close the lid, and cook until they just begin to toast, about 10 to 15 minutes. Remove the walnuts from the grill and let cool.

4. To make the pesto, in a food processor, combine walnuts, arugula, basil, Parmigiano-Reggiano, and garlic. Process until the mixture is finely chopped. With the processor running, slowly add 4 tbsp oil until well combined. Thin the pesto with 1 tbsp water (if desired). Transfer to a bowl and season with salt and pepper to taste.

5. Place salmon on the grate, close the lid, and cook until the fish reaches an internal temperature of 135°F (57°C) and just begins to flake, about 45 to 60 minutes. Remove salmon from the grill, and serve immediately with the pesto.

Grilled Fish Tacos With Peach Salsa

Servings:4

Cooking Time: 10 Minutes

Ingredients:

- 1 teaspoon cumin
- 1 teaspoon brown sugar
- 1 teaspoon ground coriander
- 2 teaspoons olive oil
- 1½ pounds fresh salmon, halibut, catfish, or your favorite fish
- Corn tortillas
- Lime wedges
- 1½ cups diced fresh peaches
- 1 firm, but ripe avocado, diced
- ¼ cup thinly sliced red onion
- 2 tablespoons chopped fresh cilantro
- ½ small jalapeño, minced
- juice of 1 lime, about 3 tablespoons

Directions:

1. Preheat the grill to 400°F using direct heat with a cast iron grate installed.
2. In a small bowl, combine cumin, sugar, and coriander. Brush fish with olive oil and sprinkle with spice mixture. Grill fish on oiled cooking grid for 3-5 minutes per side until cooked to your liking. Char tortillas on cooking grid, about 10 seconds on each side.
3. Serve tacos with fresh salsa and desired toppings. (cheese, etc.)
4. Combine salsa ingredients in a medium bowl and refrigerate until ready to use.

Cedar-plank Salmon

Servings: 4
Cooking Time: 15 Minutes

Ingredients:

- 1½lb (680g) skinless salmon, cut from the thickest part of the fish
- for the brine
- 2⁄3 cup kosher salt
- 2⁄3 cup packed light brown sugar
- 4 tbsp pickling spice
- 8 cups hot water
- for the sauce
- 2 limes
- 2 garlic cloves, minced
- 1 tbsp extra virgin olive oil
- 1 tbsp honey
- 1 tbsp soy sauce
- 1 tsp chopped fresh mint leaves, plus more to garnish
- 1-in (2.5-cm) piece ginger, peeled and grated
- kosher salt and freshly ground black pepper

Directions:

1. Place a 4 x 9in (10 x 23cm) cedar wood plank in a baking dish, cover with cold water, and place heavy cans or stones on the plank to keep it submerged. Soak for 1 to 2 hours.
2. To make the brine, in a large bowl, whisk together salt, brown sugar, pickling spice, and water until salt and sugar have dissolved. Add ice cubes a few at a time until the liquid is no longer hot. Place the salmon in a large resealable plastic bag and add brine to fully cover. (Any extra brine can be refrigerated and saved for a later use.) Refrigerate for 1 hour.
3. To make the sauce, grate the zest from 1 lime into a small bowl. Squeeze the juice of both limes and add to the bowl, then whisk in garlic, oil, honey, soy sauce, mint, and ginger. Taste and season with salt and pepper.
4. Preheat the grill to 400°F (204°C) using direct heat with a standard grate installed. Remove the cedar plank from the water and pat dry with paper towels. Place the plank on the grate until it starts to crackle and some coloring and charring appear, about 3 minutes, then turn the plank over.
5. Remove salmon from the brine and place it on the hot side of the plank. Generously brush salmon with lime sauce, close the lid, and grill until the fish is just cooked through and slightly flaky but still moist, about 12 to 15 minutes.
6. Remove salmon from the grill, lightly brush with some of the remaining sauce, and garnish with mint leaves. Serve immediately.

Marinated Grilled Salmon

Servings:4
Cooking Time: 7 Minutes

Ingredients:
- ¼ cup pineapple juice
- 2 Tablespoons soy sauce
- 2 Tablespoons brown sugar
- 1 teaspoon Kentucky Bourbon
- ¼ teaspoon black pepper
- 1/8 teaspoon garlic powder
- ½ cup vegetable oil
- 2 8oz. salmon filets
- 2 teaspoons chopped chives

Directions:
1. Preheat the grill to 350°F using direct heat with a cast iron grate installed.
2. Combine juice, soy sauce, brown sugar, bourbon, pepper, and garlic in a medium bowl. Place the fish in a shallow dish and pour the bourbon marinade over them saving a little to brush on fish as it cooks.
3. Cook fish for 5-7 minutes and regularly brush fish with marinade. Sprinkle fish with chopped chives when done.

Lemon Bed Cod

Servings: 6
Cooking Time: 15 Minutes

Ingredients:
- 6 cod filets
- 3 lemons, sliced 1/4 inch thick
- 1 onion, thinly sliced
- Salt & Pepper to taste

Directions:
1. Place lemon slices directly on the grid so they are shingled one on top of another.
2. Place onion slices on top of the lemon.
3. Grilling:
4. Preheat the grill to 400°F using direct heat with a cast iron grate installed.
5. Season both sides of the cod filets with salt and pepper and place them on top of the onion and lemon beds.
6. Close the dome for 12-15 minutes to allow the lemons to steam the fish.
7. Remove the fish on their lemon beds when the fish is opaque. Serve.

Black Pepper Dungeness Crab

Servings: 4

Cooking Time: 10 Minutes

Ingredients:

- 4 lbs Dungeness Crab
- 3 Tablespoons Hoisin sauce
- 3 Tablespoons Oyster sauce
- 2 Tablespoons butter
- 2 Tablespoons olive oil
- 2 Tablespoons freshly grated ginger
- 2 Tablespoons freshly cracked black pepper
- 2 Tablespoons red chile flakes
- 6 garlic cloves, finely chopped
- 2 green onions, finely chopped

Directions:

1. In a small sauce pan, heat butter and olive oil.
2. Add onions, garlic, ginger, pepper, and chile flakes and cook for 1 minute.
3. Add hoisin and oyster sauces and stir to warm. Keep warm over very low heat.
4. Grilling:
5. Preheat the grill to 500°F using direct heat with a cast iron grate installed.
6. Place the crabs on the grid and close the dome for 10 minutes or until the shells turn bright pink.
7. Remove the crabs from the grid and, using heat-proof gloves, quarter the crabs and slightly crack the legs.
8. Stir together half of the crabs and half of the warm sauce. Place on a platter.
9. Continue with the remaining crabs and remaining sauce. Serve

Grilled Tuna With Herb Butter

Servings:8

Cooking Time: 26minutes

Ingredients:

- 4 - 6 ounce tuna steaks
- 4 ounces herb butter (recipe follows)
- 4 bunches of Mixed Greens (Todd uses cover crop harvested from the vineyard)
- 4 breakfast radishes, shaved
- Zest and juice of 2 lemons
- 2 tablespoons olive oil
- Flake salt
- Freshly cracked black pepper
- 4 ounces Rosé dressing (recipe follows)
- 2 oz. Italian flat leaf parsley, chopped
- 1 oz. Basil, chopped
- 1 oz. Mint, chopped
- Zest of one lemon
- ¼ cup green onions, minced
- 1 stick salted butter, room temperature
- 1 teaspoon freshly ground pepper
- 3 ounces Dry Rosé wine
- 1 teaspoon superfine sugar
- 1 clove garlic minced
- 1 ounce red wine vinegar
- ¼ teaspoon dried thyme
- ¼ teaspoon freshly ground black pepper
- ½ teaspoon salt
- 4 tablespoons extra virgin olive oil

Directions:

1. Preheat the grill to 650°F using direct heat with a cast iron grate installed.

2. Season the fish with salt and pepper and grill on each side for 2-3 minutes, rotating the fish ¼ turn – halfway through the cooking on each side – to achieve beautiful cross-hatched grill lines. Once you have given the fish a ¼ turn on the second side put an ounce of the herb butter on each piece of fish and finish cooking. Fish will be a beautiful medium rare.

3. Meanwhile, in a small saucepan, combine the smashed garlic, lemon zest, juice and olive oil and heat on the grill.

4. To serve, arrange the washed cover crop on four plates, drizzle with garlic lemon oil to start the wilting process, sprinkle with sea salt and cracked pepper. Place grilled fish on top of salad. Garnish with shaved radishes and a drizzle of the rosé vinaigrette.

5. In a small bowl, combine all the ingredients and mix well. Set butter aside till ready to use.

6. Note: If you are making the butter a day in advance, pull the butter out 20 minutes before you grill the fish so it will soften slightly. Will keep in the refrigerator for 4 days.

7. In a small bowl combine the ingredients except for the oil. Once you have mixed the ingredients together, slowly whisk in the olive oil. Set dressing aside till ready to serve. Mix again just before serving.

Fish And Shrimp Stuffed Jalapeños

Servings:6

Cooking Time: 15 Minutes

Ingredients:

- Grouper
- 1 pound jalapenos
- 4-6 oz cream cheese
- 1-2 pounds shrimp
- 1 pound bacon
- Seasoning

Directions:

1. Preheat the grill to 400°F using direct heat with a cast iron grate installed.
2. Cook the grouper on a Perforated Cooking Grid. Mix with cream cheese when cooked.
3. Cut the stems off and split the jalapenos in half long ways. Use your knife to cut out the vein through the middle of the jalapeno with all the seeds. If you do not remove the seeds, your peppers will be very spicy. After removing the seeds, place the hollowed out jalapenos into your strainer and rinse them thoroughly.
4. Fill the hollowed out peppers with cream cheese and grouper. Remove the tail from your shrimp and place a single piece on top of your jalapeno. Wrap your jalapeno with half a slice of bacon and set into a Deep Dish Baking Stone.
5. Once all the jalapenos are wrapped, sprinkle with seasoning. Place jalapenos on the kamado grill for 15 minutes turning them half way through.

Scallops, Asparagus And Artichoke Gratin

Servings:6
Cooking Time: 24 Minutes

Ingredients:

- 1½ lbs U10 sea scallops
- 8 tbsp unsalted butter, divided
- ½ cup finely chopped shallots
- 6 tbsp all-purpose flour
- 2 cups cream
- 1 cup milk
- 1½ cups shaved parmesan cheese, divided
- 2 tsp kosher salt
- ½ tsp ground black pepper
- ½ tsp lemon zest
- ½ tsp crushed red pepper
- 2 pounds asparagus, trimmed and blanched
- 2 (15 ounce) cans artichoke hearts, drained
- 4 tbsp panko bread crumbs
- ½ cup crumbled bacon

Directions:

1. Preheat the grill to 400°F using direct heat with a cast iron grate installed.
2. Melt 4 tablespoons butter in a cast iron skillet; add scallops and cook until almost opaque and slightly browned, turning once. Remove from the skillet.
3. Add the remaining butter and shallots; cook, stirring occasionally about 5 minutes until tender. Stir in flour, cook for one minute. Gradually stir in milk and cream; cook 3 to 4 minutes until thickened. Stir in 1 cup cheese, salt, pepper, lemon zest and red pepper.
4. Add asparagus and artichokes, stirring to coat; cook 10 minutes. Add scallops, top with bread crumbs and bacon; cook 3 to 5 minutes more.

Grilled Shrimp And Taylor Farms Tangerine Crunch Wraps

Servings:2
Cooking Time: 6 Minutes

Ingredients:

- 1 lb. large shrimp, peeled and deveined
- Savory Pecan Seasoning
- 4-6 sundried tomato or spinach wraps
- 1 Taylor Farms Tangerine Crunch Chopped Kit
- bamboo skewers, soaked
- Feta cheese, optional

Directions:

1. Preheat the grill to 400°F using direct heat with a cast iron grate installed.
2. Season the shrimp on both sides with the Savory Pecan Seasoning. Skewer the shrimp with the soaked skewers.
3. Place the shrimp on the kamado grill and cook for 3 minutes per side or until the shrimp are pink and firm. Remove from the grill, cool and remove from the skewers.
4. Heat a plancha on the grill, griddle-side up.
5. Mix together the Taylor Farms Tangerine Crunch Chopped Kit. Fill the wrap with the salad, top with shrimp and feta cheese. Roll the wrap to enclose the salad. Heat the wrap on the plancha until you have your desired grill marks. Remove from the kamado grill and serve.

Bacon-wrapped Cod With Roasted Potatoes And Baby Arugula Salad

Servings:8

Cooking Time: 12 Minutes

Ingredients:

- 6-8 slices of thin-cut bacon
- 1 filet of cod
- 10-12 white creamer potatoes, blanched in salt water
- 2 tbsp olive oil
- Salt to taste
- 8 oz baby arugula
- 2 tbsp olive oil
- 1 lemon, zested and squeezed
- Salt to taste

Directions:

1. Preheat the grill to 400°F using direct heat with a cast iron grate installed.

2. Lay the bacon out in strips going away from you, with enough strips to cover the width of the cod. Make sure there are no gaps in the bacon. Lay the cod across the strips of bacon at the end closest to you, and roll the fish one complete turn. Tuck the ends of the bacon tightly under the roll, then continue to roll the cod away from you until you reach the end of the bacon pieces. Place the wrapped cod in a piece of plastic wrap and roll to make sure there is a tight seal. Let rest for 10 minutes.

3. Remove the cod from the plastic wrap. Using toothpicks, secure the ends of the bacon from the opposite side of the fish; you want the toothpick to just barely poke through the bacon on the seam-side, so that the fish lays flat in the skillet. Place the fish seam-side down into the cast iron skillet. While the fish is cooking, toss the potatoes in the olive oil and place directly on the grill around the cast iron skillet. Cook for about 5 minutes.

4. Remove the toothpicks from the fish and flip the fish over. Turn the potatoes to cook evenly. Cook for another 5 minutes.

5. Move the potatoes into the cast iron skillet. Remove the fish from the cast iron skillet and place directly on the grid. Cook for an additional 2 minutes, then remove the potatoes and fish from the kamado grill and let rest.

6. For the salad, mix together the baby arugula, olive oil, salt, lemon zest and lemon juice.

7. Once the fish and potatoes have cooled, cut the cod into 2-inch pieces and then smash the potatoes with palm of a hand. Top with the baby arugula salad and serve!

Red Fish Pot Pie

Servings: 6

Cooking Time: 40 Minutes

Ingredients:

- Several pounds of cubed red fish
- Potatoes
- Green Beans
- Carrots
- Onions
- Cream of asparagus soup
- French fried onions
- Crescent rolls

Directions:

1. Preheat the grill to 350°F using direct heat with a cast iron grate installed. Meanwhile, inside, boil the potatoes, green beans, carrots and onions.

2. Place cubes of red fish in a greased 9 x 13" pan. Pour the boiled veggies (drained of water) onto the fish. Pour the cream of asparagus soup on top and spread around with a rubber spatula. Layer on the French fried onions.

3. To make dough – roll out the crescent rolls on a clean surface and lay it on top of the other ingredients in the pan.

4. Bake for 30-40 minutes.

5. Remove from grill. You can allow to rest for a few minutes if you like, or consume immediately.

Florida Lobster Roll

Servings:6
Cooking Time: 28 Minutes

Ingredients:

- 4 tablespoons butter, divided
- Garlic powder
- 3 Florida lobster tails, about 7 ounces each
- ½ cup mayonnaise
- Zest from ½ of a Florida orange
- 1/3 cup finely chopped celery
- Pinch dried tarragon
- 6 hot dog buns, top split if available
- Slices of Florida avocado
- Spinach leaves

Directions:

1. Preheat the grill to 350°F using direct heat with a cast iron grate installed.
2. Split the top of the lobster shells and pull the meat out to rest on top. Cut a few slits in the meat so the lobster will cook evenly (you can have your fish monger do this for you). Place the tails on a perforated cooking grid and season lightly with salt and pepper.
3. Melt two tablespoons of butter and mix in a pinch of garlic powder. Brush the tails liberally with the butter. Place in the kamado grill and cook until the tails are firm to the touch, about 25 minutes; remove and let cool.
4. Remove the platesetter to cook direct at 350°F/177°C. Melt the remaining butter and mix in a pinch of garlic powder. Brush the sides of the rolls and grill them for 2 to 3 minutes on each side until golden brown. Remove the lobster meat from the shells and cut into large dice. Add to the dressing and mix well. Line each bun with a few spinach leaves. Lay a few slices of avocado in the bun and top each with an equal portion of the lobster mix.
5. Mix ingredients together in a large bowl.

Grilled Lobster Tails

Servings:4
Cooking Time:6 Minutes

Ingredients:

- 4 (4-ounce) lobster tails, cleaned
- 1 tablespoon Better Than Bouillon Lobster Base
- 1 cup softened, unsalted butter
- 1 tablespoon sambel oelek (Fresh chili paste)
- 1/4 cup freshly chopped parsley
- 1 teaspoon Better Than Bouillon Roasted Garlic Base

Directions:

1. Preheat the grill to 450°F using direct heat with a cast iron grate installed.
2. Mix the Lobster Base, butter, fresh chili paste, parsley, and Roasted Garlic Base in a small bowl. Divide the butter in half.
3. Spread 2 tablespoons of the butter over the meat of each lobster tail. Place the lobsters directly onto the kamado grill, meat side up, and grill for 5-6 minutes.
4. Melt the remaining reserved butter. Remove lobsters from kamado grill and serve immediately with the remaining butter.

Hatch Chili Shrimp And Grits

Servings:8

Cooking Time: 27 Minutes

Ingredients:

- 2 cups uncooked grits
- 4 cups water
- ½ tbsp salt
- 6 tbsp unsalted butter, divided
- 1 tsp black pepper
- 3 cups shredded cheddar cheese
- 6 cloves garlic, minced on a microplane
- ¼ cup chopped cilantro
- 2 scallions, chopped
- 2 lbs deveined shrimp, tails off
- 8 slices bacon
- 2 tbsp Ancho Chili & Coffee Seasoning
- 8 Hatch Chilies

Directions:

1. Preheat the grill to 450°F using direct heat with a cast iron grate installed.

2. Lightly salt the water (1/4 tbsp) and add to the dutch oven; place the dutch oven on the grid while prepping and bring to a boil. Add the grits and 2 tablespoons of butter, stirring to incorporate all ingredients. Cook for 5-10 minutes, or until all of the water has disappeared. Add cheese, garlic, cilantro, ¼ tbsp salt, black pepper and the rest of the butter. Mix thoroughly and set aside.

3. Put the cast iron skillet in the middle of the kamado grill to heat. Around it, place your Hatch chilies for roasting. Roast them until the outer skin is blistered and dark, then place them in a resealable bag to steam for 10-15 minutes. Carefully peel the outer layer of skin off and discard; remove the seeds and discard. Chop the remaining chilies and put in a bowl.

4. While the chilies are roasting, cook the bacon in the skillet until it is crispy, remove, chop and set aside. In the bacon grease, add the shrimp and season with Ancho Chili & Coffee Seasoning. Cook 2 minutes per side, remove and set aside.

5. Remove the skillet from the kamado grill, making sure to stir the contents at the bottom. Add your grits in an even layer spread across the bottom of the skillet. Add bacon, shrimp, scallions and chopped Hatch Chilies. Enjoy!

Cedar-planked Salmon

Servings:4
Cooking Time: 15 Minutes

Ingredients:

- 2 tablespoons extra-virgin olive oil
- ½ cup Dijon mustard
- ¼ cup honey
- 1 tablespoon balsamic vinegar
- 2 teaspoons grated orange zest
- 1 teaspoon minced fresh thyme plus extra for garnish
- 4 (7-ounce) salmon fillets, skin on
- Kosher salt and freshly ground black pepper
- 2 cedar planks

Directions:

1. Preheat the grill to 400°F using direct heat with a cast iron grate installed.
2. Place the cedar planks in a pan, cover with water, and let soak for 1 hour.
3. Whisk the mustard, honey, balsamic vinegar, orange zest, and 1 teaspoon thyme together in a small bowl.
4. Place the cedar planks on the grid, close the lid of the grill, and preheat for 3 minutes. Open the lid and turn the planks over, brush them with the olive oil, and place 2 salmon fillets on each plank. Season the salmon with salt and pepper and brush generously with the honey glaze. Close the lid of the grill. Cook the salmon for 12 to 15 minutes for medium.
5. Remove from the heat, garnish with thyme, and serve immediately.

Greek Sea Bass

Servings: 4
Cooking Time: 15 Minutes

Ingredients:

- 2 whole sea bass (approximately 1 pound each), cleaned and gutted
- 1/4 cup olive oil
- 2 Tablespoons lemon juice
- 2 Tablespoons capers
- 2 Tablespoons parsley, chopped
- 1 tsp fresh oregano, chopped
- 1/2 tsp salt
- 1/4 tsp dried chili flakes
- 4 cloves garlic
- 1 lemon, thinly sliced

Directions:

1. Whisk together herbs, lemon juice, capers, olive oil, salt, and chili flakes. Set aside.
2. Season the sea bass with salt and pepper on the inside cavity and place lemon slices inside.
3. Grilling:
4. Preheat the grill to 400°F using direct heat with a cast iron grate installed.
5. Place whole fish on the grid and close the dome for 6 minutes.
6. Gently flip the fish and replace the dome for an additional 6-8 minutes or until the fish is cooked through.
7. Remove the sea bass and drizzle with herb and lemon mixture. Serve more on the side for dressing as the fish is eaten.

Grilled Caribbean Snapper With Vera Cruz Salsa

Servings:4

Cooking Time: 16 Minutes

Ingredients:

- 2 Second City Snapper filets
- 1½ tbsp paprika
- 1 tbsp white vinegar
- ¾ tsp dried oregano
- 1 garlic clove, minced
- ¼ tsp cumin
- Juice of 2 limes
- Splash of olive oil
- 1 red bell pepper
- 5 mini sweet peppers
- 2 serrano chilies
- 5 plum tomatoes
- Olive oil for brushing the veggies
- Coarsely ground salt and pepper
- 1 cup pitted Manzanilla olives, chopped
- ¼ cup fresh chopped cilantro
- 1 tbsp capers, drained
- 1 tsp fresh thyme leaves
- 1 tsp Mexican oregano
- 2 tbsp red wine vinegar
- ¼ cup extra virgin olive oil
- Juice of 1 lime

Directions:

1. One day before the cook, combine all the seasoning paste ingredients in a small bowl until well blended and smooth. Refrigerate until ready to cook.

2. Preheat the grill to 400°F using direct heat with a cast iron grate installed.

3. Rub each side of the filet generously with the seasoning paste. Grill the fish directly on the cooking grid until the paste is nicely charred – 5-7 minutes on each side until the internal temperature reaches a minimum of 145°F. Transfer the fish to a platter, spoon salsa on top and garnish with fresh herbs.

4. For the salsa, brush the peppers, chilies and tomatoes with olive oil; season with salt and pepper. Grill until slightly charred on all sides, about 2 minutes per side. Remove to a bowl, cover with plastic wrap and let steam for 10 minutes or so. Remove the skins and seeds and dice. Combine the diced peppers, tomatoes, chilies and all other ingredients in a bowl and let mixture sit at room temperature for 30 minutes allowing the flavors to meld.

Herb Butter Lobster Tails

Servings: 4
Cooking Time: 10 Minutes

Ingredients:
- 4 lobster tails, cut in half
- 1 recipe Compound Herb Butter flavored with lemon zest, tarragon, parsley, and garlic

Directions:
1. Place 1 Tablespoon of Compound Herb Butter on top of each lobster tail half.
2. Grilling:
3. Preheat the grill to 500°F using direct heat with a cast iron grate installed.
4. Place the tails directly on the grid and close the dome for 10 minutes.
5. Carefully remove the lobster tails taking care not to spill any of the butter and serve with crusty bread.

Ginger Scallion Scallops

Servings: 4
Cooking Time: 7 Minutes

Ingredients:
- 1 lb large sea scallops
- 1/4 cup chopped green onion
- 2 Tablespoons fresh orange juice
- 2 tsp sesame oil
- 1 tsp honey
- 1 tsp freshly grated ginger
- 1/2 tsp sriracha

Directions:
1. Combine onion, orange juice, sesame oil, honey, ginger and sriracha in a shallow dish.
2. Allow the scallops to marinate 3 minutes on each side.
3. Grilling:
4. Preheat the grill to 425°F using direct heat with a cast iron grate installed.
5. Place the scallops on the grid and close the dome for 3 minutes.
6. If the scallops turn easily, flip them and close the dome for another 2-4 minutes.

Country Ham, Shrimp & Grits Kabobs

Servings:8

Cooking Time: 67 Minutes

Ingredients:

- 1 cup grits
- 1 cup shredded cheddar
- ¼ cup Oliver Farms Pecan Oil or Butter
- 1 cup country ham, fine dice
- ½ cup diced scallions
- ½ cup red pepper, fine dice
- ½ cup yellow pepper, fine dice
- 1 cup heavy cream
- 4 cups water
- 2 tsp salt
- ½ tsp black pepper
- ½ tsp dried thyme
- 1 pound 26-30 count shrimp, peeled and deveined, tail on
- ¼ cup olive oil
- 1 Tbsp Dijon mustard
- 1 tsp minced garlic
- 2 Tbsp fresh lemon juice
- Salt and pepper
- 1 red pepper, seeded, membrane removed, cut in 1" squares
- 1 yellow pepper, seeded, membrane removed, cut in 1" squares
- 1 red onion, peeled, cut in 1" squares, separate layers

Directions:

1. Cook diced ham in butter or oil until almost crisp. Add diced peppers and scallions. Cook until soft. Add cream, water and spices. Bring to a boil, gradually stir in grits. Bring back to a boil, then lower to simmer. Continue cooking for 45-60 minutes, adding a little more liquid if needed; they need to be thick. Remove from heat and stir in cheese until melted. Pour into greased 9" x 13" pan. Chill overnight.

2. Combine olive oil, Dijon, garlic, lemon juice, salt and pepper in a bowl. Add shrimp to mixture and marinate about 30 minutes

3. Cut grits into 1 square. Broil in oven on both sides until golden. Thread wooden skewers with 1 grits cube then pierce one piece each of red pepper, yellow pepper and red onion. Chill until ready to use.

4. Preheat the grill to 350°F using direct heat with a cast iron grate installed. Place skewers on the cooking grid; close dome and cook 5-7 minutes or until shrimp are opaque. Use spatula to carefully lift from underneath.

POULTRY

Grill Glazed Sweet Asian Chicken Pan Grill

Servings: 4

Cooking Time: 15 Minutes

Ingredients:

- 3 chicken breasts, cut into bite-size pieces
- 2 cups broccoli, cut into bite-size pieces
- 1 red bell pepper, cut into thin 1" strips
- 1 medium red onion, cut into thin 1" strips
- 1 yellow bell pepper, cut into thin 1" strips
- 1 tablespoon soy sauce
- 1⁄4 cup brown sugar
- 1⁄2 tablespoon Better Than Bouillon Chicken Base
- 1⁄2 teaspoon fresh ginger, finely chopped
- 1⁄4 cup water

Directions:

1. Preheat the grill to 450°F using direct heat with a cast iron grate installed.
2. In a bowl, mix soy sauce, brown sugar, Roasted Chicken Base, ginger and water.
3. Mix chicken and all vegetables in a Stir-Fry and Paella Pan. Place on the kamado grill.
4. Cook approximately 12-15 minutes or until chicken is thoroughly cooked and vegetables are soft.
5. Serve with rice or Asian noodles.

Brined Roasted Turkey

Servings:4
Cooking Time: 240 Minutes

Ingredients:

- 4 qts water
- 1 ½ cup kosher salt
- ½ cup sugar
- 2 bay leaves
- 2 tbsp black peppercorns
- 1 tbsp dried sage
- 1 orange, cut in half
- 1 lemon, cut in half
- 1 onion, cut in half
- 8 cloves of garlic
- Enough ice to fill the bottom of the brining bucket about 3 inches

- 1 12-14 lb. whole turkey
- 1 orange, cut into wedges
- 1 sweet onion, cut into wedges
- 1 lemon, cut into wedges
- 2 whole heads of garlic, top cut off
- 3 sprigs rosemary
- 3 sprigs thyme
- 3 sprigs sage
- Savory Pecan Seasoning
- Extra virgin olive oil or canola oil
- Kosher salt

Directions:

1. A day before your cook, put all the brine ingredients, except for ice, into a pot and boil for 10 minutes. Pour liquid over ice into the brining bucket. Once the liquid is cool place the turkey into the bucket, making sure the turkey is completely submerged. Cover tightly, and put into the fridge and brine for 8-24 hours. When ready to cook, remove the turkey from the brine and rinse thoroughly.

2. Preheat the grill to 350°F using direct heat with a cast iron grate installed.

3. Pat the turkey dry and coat with oil, season with salt and Savory Pecan Seasoning.

4. Place half of the onion, one whole head of garlic, half the orange, half the lemon, and two sprigs of each herb inside the cavity of the turkey. Fold the wings back behind the turkey so that they cook evenly. Put the turkey on the roasting rack and place into the drip pan. Add the remaining garlic, onion, orange, lemon and herbs around the turkey in the drip pan.

5. Place on the kamado grill and cook 3-4 hours or until the internal temperature is 165°F (white meat) and 185°F (dark meat). During the cook, cover the turkey with aluminum foil once the skin has the desired color and texture.

6. Remove from the kamado grill, let rest for 15 minutes. Carve and enjoy!

Grilled Hot Candy Chicken Wings

Servings:4
Cooking Time: 30 Minutes

Ingredients:

- 5 pounds Springer Mountain Farms Chicken Wings split chicken wings, rinsed and dried
- ¼ cup Sweet & Smoky Seasoning
- 2 tbsp seasoned salt
- 2 tbsp cooking oil
- 2 cups Kansas City Style BBQ Sauce
- ½ cup hot sauce
- 1 cup honey
- ½ cup ground cinnamon

Directions:

1. Preheat the grill to 350°F using direct heat with a cast iron grate installed with hickory wood chips. Grill for about 30 minutes or until the internal temperature reached 165°F or higher. Turn the wings occasionally for even cooking.
2. For the dry rub, mix the barbecue rub and seasoned salt into a bowl and blend well. Place the chicken wings in a large resealable plastic bag. Pour in the dry rub and oil, shake to coat the wings well. Marinate overnight in the refrigerator.
3. For the Hot Candy Sauce, mix the ingredients well. Coat the cooked wings with the sauce and serve.

Grilled Pheasant With Chimichurri

Servings: 4
Cooking Time: 30 Minutes

Ingredients:

- 2 pheasants (about 1 1/4 to 1 1/2 pounds each)
- 4 cups Turkey Brine
- 1 cup Chimichurri

Directions:

1. Cover pheasants with Turkey Brine and allow to sit a minimum of 2 hours or up to overnight.
2. Grilling:
3. Preheat the grill to 400°F using direct heat with a cast iron grate installed. Put the plate setter in place along with the grid.
4. Place the dried pheasants on the grid and cover for 30 minutes or until the internal temperature of the thigh reaches 160°F.
5. Remove the pheasants from the grill and cover with chimichurri. Serve.

Bbq Chicken Cheddar Sandwich

Servings:4

Cooking Time: 35 Minutes

Ingredients:

- 4 slices of Nature's Own 12-Grain Bread
- 2 cups thinly sliced red onion
- 2 teaspoons brown sugar
- 1/8 teaspoon salt
- 1/4 teaspoon dried thyme leaves
- 2 cups shredded cooked chicken breast
- 3 tablespoons BBQ sauce
- 2 teaspoons vegetable oil
- 4 (1-ounce) slices reduced-fat deli-style Cheddar cheese

Directions:

1. Preheat the grill to 350°F using direct heat with a cast iron grate installed.

2. Cook chicken 10-12 minutes per side, then toss in bowl with barbecue sauce until evenly coated.

3. Heat oil in Stir-Fry and Paella Pan.

4. Add onion, brown sugar and thyme; cook 10 minutes or until onion is tender and lightly browned, stirring often. Remove from heat; stir in salt. Set aside.

5. Divide chicken and onion evenly over bread slices; top each with 1 cheese slice. Wrap each open-faced sandwich in heavy-duty foil forming a loose packet; seal all edges.

6. Add to cooking grid for 8 minutes or until heated through. Carefully open foil packets and drizzle with additional barbecue sauce, if desired.

Green Tomato Pizza With Smoked Chicken And Truffle Crema

Servings:8

Cooking Time: 10 Minutes

Ingredients:

- 8 oz (227 g) smoked chicken or turkey, pulled
- ½ red bell pepper, slivered
- 8 oz (227 g) fresh mozzarella cheese, cut into thin slices
- 2 tbsp (30 ml) fresh corn kernels (drain well if using canned)
- 4 or 5 fresh basil leaves, lightly chopped
- 1 cup (240 ml) warm water
- 1 tsp (5 ml) sugar
- 1 tsp (5 ml) active dry yeast
- 3 cups (710 ml) all-purpose flour
- 1½ tsp (8 ml) kosher salt
- ½ tsp (3 ml) dried Italian seasoning (optional)
- 2 tsp (10 ml) olive oil, divided
- 2 tbsp (30 ml) olive oil
- 5 medium green tomatoes
- ½ cup (120 ml) thinly sliced sweet or white onion
- 2 cloves garlic, minced
- 1 tsp (5 ml) kosher salt
- ½ tsp (3 ml) freshly ground black pepper
- 1 tsp (5 ml) sugar
- 1 tbsp (15 ml) white vinegar
- 2 tsp (10 ml) hot red pepper flakes
- ¼ cup (60 ml) fresh basil leaves, roughly chopped
- 1 tsp (5 ml) diced fresh oregano
- ½ cup (120 ml) crema
- 1½ tsp (8 ml) white truffle olive oil

Directions:

1. Run warm water until it is around 110°F, then measure 1 cup (240 ml) into a small bowl. Add the sugar and whisk, then sprinkle in the yeast and let sit until it blooms, 5 to 10 minutes.

2. With a stand mixer, mix together the flour, salt and Italian seasoning. Pour in the water/yeast and blend on low speed until combined. Add 1 tsp (5ml) of the olive oil and continue to blend until a dough forms, then keep mixing for 5 or 6 minutes. Lightly flour a Dough Rolling Mat, dump the dough onto it, and form into a ball. Drizzle the remaining teaspoon of olive oil into a large mixing bowl to coat the inside of the bowl. Transfer the dough ball to the bowl, cover with a damp towel, and let rise until it doubles in size, about 1½ hours.

3. While the dough is rising, prepare the sauce. Use 1 tsp (5 ml) of the olive oil to lightly oil the green tomatoes and char on the kamado grill, then set aside. In a small stockpot over medium heat, heat the remaining olive oil, add the onion and cook until softened, 3 to 4 minutes. Then add the garlic and cook for 2 minutes. Core and chop the tomatoes and add them along with the salt, pepper, sugar, vinegar and red pepper. Cook for 5 minutes, then decrease the heat and simmer for 25 to 30 minutes, stirring occasionally, until the tomatoes are soft. Stir in the basil and oregano, then, using an immersion blender (or food processor), blend until smooth.

4. To make the truffle crema, whisk the crema and truffle oil together. Store covered in the refrigerator until needed.

5. When the dough has risen, place on a lightly floured Dough Rolling Mat and knead 4 or 5 times, then divide into 4 parts. Roll out each piece into a 10 in (25 cm) circle (the thinner the better).

6. To assemble, spoon ½ cup (120 ml) sauce onto each crust and spread with the bottom of a spoon. Lay fresh mozzarella cheese on the pizza, then sprinkle smoked chicken, red bell pepper and fresh corn kernels over the pizzas.

7. Preheat the grill to 600°F using direct heat with a cast iron grate installed. Add a Pizza & Baking Stone. Dust a Pizza Peel with cornmeal, add a pizza, and slide onto the Stone for 5 to 6 minutes, or until the crust is browned and any cheese is melted. Remove and drizzle the Truffle Crema over the pizza, using a fork. Then sprinkle on the basil and serve.

Chicken Cacciatore

Servings: 4
Cooking Time: 40 Minutes

Ingredients:

- 4 lbs chicken thighs, bone in and skin on
- 1/4 cup freshly chopped basil
- 3 cloves garlic, minced
- 1 bell pepper, sliced
- 1 onion, sliced
- 3/4 cups dry white wine
- 3/4 cups chicken stock
- 1/2 cup flour
- 3 Tablespoons olive oil
- 3 Tablespoons capers
- 1 1/2 tsp dried oregano
- 1 (28 ounce) can diced tomatoes with juice
- Salt and Pepper

Directions:

1. Preheat the grill to 500°F using direct heat with a cast iron grate installed with the dutch oven on the grid.
2. Season each chicken piece with salt and pepper and lightly dredge in flour.
3. Place olive oil in the dutch oven and brown chicken pieces on all sides. Work in batches and set chicken aside.
4. Drain all but 2 Tablespoon of the fat in the dutch oven and add onion, garlic, and bell pepper and cook until soft.
5. Add chicken back into the pot and add wine and chicken stock, scraping the bottom of the dutch oven.
6. Add tomatoes, oregano and capers, stir and cover.
7. Reduce the heat in the grill to 400°F and lower the dome for 35 minutes.
8. Garnish with fresh basil and serve.

Jerk Chicken Wings

Servings:4
Cooking Time: 20 Minutes

Ingredients:

- 2 pounds chicken wings, tips removed
- 2 Tablespoons Better Than Bouillon Organic Chicken Base
- 1/4 cup Jerk seasoning
- 1/4 cup apple cider vinegar
- 1 Tablespoon garlic powder

Directions:

1. Mix the chicken base, Jerk seasoning, vinegar, and garlic powder in a small bowl. Add the marinade and chicken wings to a re-sealable plastic bag. Toss to coat and place in the refrigerator for 2 hours and up to 8 hours.
2. Preheat the grill to 450°F using direct heat with a cast iron grate installed.
3. Remove the chicken wings from the marinade and place directly onto kamado grill. Grill the wings for 10 minutes per side. Remove the wings from the kamado grill and serve immediately.

Wild Rice Turkey Biryani Stuffed Whole Pumpkin

Servings:12

Cooking Time: 40 Minutes

Ingredients:

- 1 large sugar pumpkin (approx. 3-4 pounds)
- 6 tbsp clarified butter
- 2 sweet onions, chopped
- 3 cloves garlic, minced
- 1 tsp fresh ginger, minced
- 10 green cardamom pods
- 3 whole cinnamon sticks
- ¼ tsp ground cloves
- ¼ tsp chili powder
- 1 tsp ground cumin
- 1 tsp ground coriander
- ½ tsp ground black pepper
- 1 cup wild rice
- 1 cup basmati rice, rinsed until clear water
- 2 lbs. ground turkey or chicken, cooked and browned
- 1 lemon
- 1 cup Craisins
- 1 cup tart apple (Granny Smith), diced
- ¾ cup pecans, toasted and chopped
- Coconut Oil
- Dizzy Pig Curry-ish
- 4 cups water

Directions:

1. Prepare Pumpkin:
2. Wash and dry the pumpkin.
3. Slice the top off the pumpkin using a sharp knife.
4. Remove the seeds and stringy center. Save the seeds for later.
5. Rub the inside of the pumpkin with melted coconut oil and Dizzy Pig Curry-ish.
6. Prepare Biryani (can be made a day ahead):
7. Melt the butter in a dutch oven.
8. Add the chopped onion and cook until browned.
9. Add garlic and ginger and next 7 ingredients. Saute until the spices "bloom", but careful not to burn.
10. Add the wild rice and basmati rice and mix well.
11. Add the water to the rice mixture and bring to a boil, cover and simmer for 30 minutes or until all of the liquid has been absorbed. Remove from heat.
12. Remove cinnamon sticks and cardamom pods from mixture.
13. Add the turkey, juice of 1 lemon, Craisins, apple and pecans.
14. Prepare Egg & Pumpkin:
15. Preheat the grill to 325°F using direct heat with a cast iron grate installed.
16. Place pumpkin in a pie plate.
17. Fill pumpkin to top with Biryani and place pumpkin lid on top.

18. Place pumpkin in pie plate on the platesetter – preferable to use the egg "feet" to raise it off the platesetter, but can be put directly on it.

19. Close lid of the egg and be sure that the stem of the pumpkin clears the hole on the Egg lid and that the temperature gauge does not pierce the flesh of the Egg.

20. Roast the pumpkin for 40 minutes or until a toothpick or knife can be inserted with minimal resistance. It should be the consistency of a cooked baked potato.

21. Remove from Egg and allow to rest with the top on for at least 10 minutes.

22. To Serve:

23. Scoop out the Biryani, ensuring to scoop the roasted pumpkin in the serving. Enjoy!

Wasabi Honey Teriyaki Grilled Chicken Thighs

Servings:4
Cooking Time: 16 Minutes

Ingredients:

- 2 tsp (10mL) wasabi powder
- 2 tsp (10mL) freshly squeezed lemon juice
- 1 oz (30mL) sake
- 1/2 cup (125mL) honey
- 1 tbsp (15mL) soy sauce
- 3 tbsp (45mL) hoisin sauce
- 1 tsp (5mL) prepared horseradish, drained of excess moisture
- 1 tsp (5mL) minced ginger
- 1 green onion, minced
- 12 boneless skinless chicken thighs
- Kosher salt and freshly ground black pepper to taste
- Pinch of cinnamon
- 1/4 cup (60mL) crushed wasabi peas
- 1 tsp (5mL) toasted sesame seeds
- 1 tbsp (15mL) chopped fresh cilantro

Directions:

1. Place the wasabi powder into a small bowl and drizzle with the lemon juice and sake. Stir in honey, soy sauce, hoisin sauce, horseradish, ginger and green onion.
2. Preheat the grill to 450°F using direct heat with a cast iron grate installed.
3. Season both sides of the thighs with kosher salt, black pepper and a pinch of cinnamon.
4. Grill the thighs for 6-8 minutes on one side, turn the thighs over and begin to baste with the wasabi honey baste. Continue to cook for another 6-8 minutes, basting with the sauce until fully cooked, minimum internal temperature of 160°F. Remove from kamado grill.
5. Sprinkle with crushed wasabi peas, toasted sesame seeds and fresh cilantro. Serve immediately.

Greg Bates Bbq Chicken

Servings:8
Cooking Time: 30 Minutes

Ingredients:

- Trimmed chicken Breasts
- 2 cups Dr Pepper
- 2 cups ketchup
- 1/2 cup no-pulp orange juice
- 1/4 cup Worcestershire sauce
- 1/4 cup molasses
- 1 tsp ground ginger
- 1 tsp hot paprika
- 1 tsp chipotle Chile powder
- 2 tsp garlic powder
- 2 tsp onion powder
- 1/2 teaspoon crushed red pepper flakes

Directions:

1. Preheat the grill to 450°F using direct heat with a cast iron grate installed.
2. On your grill over medium high heat for 10 to 15 minutes on each side, brushing the Dr Pepper BBQ sauce on the chicken each time you turn it over. Grill until chicken is cooked through and juices run clear.
3. Mix the Dr Pepper, ketchup, orange juice, Worcestershire sauce and molasses in a saucepan. Season with paprika, ginger, garlic powder, red pepper flakes, chipotle powder and onion powder. Bring the sauce to a boil over high heat, proceed to reduce to medium-low heat and simmer for 15 minutes while stirring occasionally.
4. Use right away on your BBQ chicken, or store in your fridge for about a week! Enjoy.

Vidalia Onion And Sriracha-glazed Nashville Hot Wings

Servings:4

Cooking Time: 35 Minutes

Ingredients:

- 1 pound whole chicken wings
- 1 tbsp olive oil
- Nashville Hot Seasoning, to taste
- ½ bottle of Vidalia Onion and Sriracha Sauce

Directions:

1. Preheat the grill to 350°F using direct heat with a cast iron grate installed.
2. Separate the flats from the drumettes, discarding the wing tips. Coat with the olive oil and a generous amount of the Nashville Hot Seasoning.
3. Place the wings skin-side down on the grid and cook for 15 minutes. Flip the wings after 15 minutes and cook for another 15-20 minutes, or until the wings measure 175°F internally. Remove the wings and place in a bowl.
4. Pour in ½ bottle of the Vidalia Onion and Sriracha Sauce and stir to coat the wings while they are still hot. Serve and enjoy!

Rathbun Chicken

Servings:

Cooking Time: Minutes

Ingredients:

- 6 pound chicken
- Your favorite poultry seasoning
- Chicken thighs or breast
- Maple spice

Directions:

1. Preheat the grill to 325°F using direct heat with a cast iron grate installed.
2. In a roasting pan, season chicken by pouring spices inside the chicken and rubbing the outside as well.
3. Place chicken directly on the grid and cook to internal temperature of 172-175°F.
4. Place breast or thighs in the roasting pan and season with maple spices and place directly on the grid. Cook to same internal temperature as the whole chicken.
5. The chicken is ready when the juices run clear.

Butter-injected Turkey And Sides

Servings:16
Cooking Time: 350 Minutes

Ingredients:

- 1 12-14 lb. whole turkey
- 5 oz. Roasted Garlic & Herb Banner Butter, melted
- 1 orange, cut into wedges
- 1 sweet onion, cut into wedges
- 1 lemon, cut into wedges
- 2 whole heads of garlic, top cut off
- 3 sprigs rosemary
- 3 sprigs thyme
- 3 sprigs sage
- Savory Pecan Seasoning
- Extra virgin olive oil or canola oil
- Kosher salt
- 6 whole carrots
- ½ lb. red potatoes cut in half
- 8 oz whole baby Portobello mushrooms
- 2 zucchinis, cut into ½ inch strips
- 8 oz cherry tomatoes
- 8 oz green beans
- 5 oz. Fig & Balsamic Banner Butter, melted
- 2 tbsp extra virgin olive oil
- ½ tbsp kosher salt
- ¼ tbsp cracked black pepper
- 2 tbsp Worcestershire sauce
- 4 sweet potatoes
- 2 tbsp brown sugar
- ½ tbsp kosher salt
- ½ cup butter

Directions:

1. Preheat the grill to 350°F using direct heat with a cast iron grate installed.
2. Pat the turkey dry and coat with oil, season with salt and Savory Pecan Seasoning. Pull melted butter into the injector and evenly inject the turkey with the butter (to prevent splash back from the injector, cover the turkey with plastic wrap and inject the turkey through the plastic wrap.)
3. Place half of the onion, one whole head of garlic, half the orange, half the lemon, and two sprigs of each herb inside the cavity of the turkey. Fold the wings back behind the turkey so that they cook evenly. Add the remaining garlic, onion, orange, lemon and herbs around the turkey in the drip pan.
4. Place on the grill and cook 3-4 hours or until the internal temperature is 165°F (white meat) and 185°F (dark meat). During the cook, cover the turkey with aluminum foil once the skin has the desired color and texture.
5. Remove from the grill, let rest for 15 minutes. Carve and enjoy!
6. Preheat the grill to 350°F using direct heat with a cast iron grate installed.
7. Coat the dutch oven lid with extra virgin olive oil. Place all vegetables into the dutch oven lid. In a bowl, mix melted butter, Worcestershire sauce, pepper and salt. Pour evenly over the top of the vegetables.
8. Roast for 45 minutes, remove from the grill and serve.
9. Preheat the grill to 350°F using direct heat with a cast iron grate installed.
10. Poke holes in the sweet potato, all over. Bake until soft and skin has blistered – about 50 minutes to an hour.
11. Remove from the grill and let rest for 10 minutes. Peel the skin off and discard. Place in a bowl and mash the sweet potatoes. Add salt, and butter and mix thoroughly. Enjoy!

Green Curry Chicken

Servings: 4

Cooking Time: 40 Minutes

Ingredients:

- 2 lbs boneless skinless chicken breast, cut into 1 inch cubes
- 1 Tablespoon garlic, minced
- 1 Tablespoon ginger, grated
- 2 green onions, chopped
- 2 cups unsweetened coconut milk
- 2 Tablespoon canola oil
- 2 Tablespoon soy sauce
- 2 Tablespoons cornstarch
- 2 Tablespoons Thai green curry paste
- 2 Tablespoons brown sugar
- 1 Tablespoon fish sauce

Directions:

1. Preheat the grill to 500°F using direct heat with a cast iron grate installed with the dutch oven on the grid.
2. Dredge chicken breast pieces in soy sauce, then corn starch.
3. Place oil and chicken in the heated dutch oven and brown. Work in batches, being careful not to overcrowd the pan.
4. Add garlic, ginger, and green onion and stir until fragrant.
5. Add Thai green curry paste, fish sauce, coconut milk, and sugar and stir to combine.
6. Lower the temperature in the grill to 350°F.
7. Cover the dutch oven and the dome and simmer for 25-30 minutes.
8. Serve over jasmine rice with lime wedges and whole cilantro leaves.

Smokey Thai Pulled Chicken Sandwiches

Servings:6

Cooking Time: 92 Minutes

Ingredients:

- 3 lbs boneless skinless chicken thighs
- 1 package of Cobblestone Bread Co.™ Sesame Twist Hamburger Rolls
- 3 tbs chopped cilantro
- quick pickled carrots
- * optional Sriracha sauce
- 3 cups water
- 2 tbs pure cane sugar
- juice of one lime
- 2 tsp Thai fish sauce
- 2 tsp soy sauce
- 1 tbs sea salt
- 1-2 hot peppers (Thai bird or Serrano)
- 2 cloves of garlic
- 1 tbs pure cane sugar
- 2 tsp sea salt
- 1 tsp onion powder
- ½ tsp ground ginger
- ½ tsp garlic powder
- ¼ tsp ground white pepper
- ¼ cup water
- ¼ cup honey
- 1 tbs fresh lime juice
- 2 tbs soy sauce
- 1 tsp Thai fish sauce (add while mixing, do not heat)
- ⅔ pound carrots
- 2½ cups water
- ⅔ cup rice wine vinegar
- 1 tbs pure cane sugar
- 2 tsp sea salt
- 2 tsp fresh grated ginger

Directions:

1. Whisk together ingredients for the brine. Add the chicken thighs, making sure they are fully covered. Place in refrigerator for 2-3 hours.

2. About a half hour before you are ready to grill.Preheat the grill to 280°F using direct heat with a cast iron grate installed.

3. Whisk together the dry rub ingredients. Remove the chicken thighs from brine, and pat dry. Discard brine. Generously coat the chicken with dry rub.

4. Place chicken thighs on the kamado grill. Cook for 1½ hours, flipping once after about 50 minutes. Check temperature occasionally to make sure you are not gout over a maximum of 325°F, damper more narrowly to reduce temperature closer to 280°F.

5. Prepare the Quick Pickled Carrots while the chicken is grilling.

6. When chicken thighs are removed from the kamado grill, set aside to rest and cool a little, then pull the chicken (discard any fatty bits). Mix in chopped fresh cilantro.

7. Mix sauce ingredients, except fish sauce, in a small saucepan over medium-high heat. Once it comes to a boil, reduce to a simmer. Allow to gently bubble for 2 minutes, then shut off and pour over the pulled chicken. Mix. Add fish sauce and mix again.

8. Place some of the pickled matchstick carrots on the bottom half of each Cobblestone Bread Co.™ Sesame Twist Hamburger Roll. Top with a generous helping of the Thai pulled chicken (squirt on a bit of sriracha sauce if you like) and cover with top of the roll.

9. Peel and trim carrots, then matchstick slice.

10. Whisk together pickling brine ingredients in a deep microwave-safe bowl. Microwave for 2 minutes, then whisk again to ensure salt & sugar are dissolved. Add the carrots. Make sure they are fully covered in the brine.

11. Microwave until the brine come to a quick boil (about 5-6 minutes). Microwave for another minute (you may need to stop it a couple times to avoid boil over). Remove from the microwave and set aside to cool.

12. When the brine has cooled to room temperature, drain. Refrigerate the carrots until ready to go on sandwiches.

Bbq Chicken Soup

Servings: 8

Cooking Time: 35 Minutes

Ingredients:

- 12 ounces applewood-smoked bacon, diced (about 14 slices)
- 4 tablespoons of your favorite barbecue seasoning
- 1½ pounds tomatoes, chopped (about 4 cups)
- 1½ cups chopped yellow onions
- ¼ cup minced garlic
- 1 chipotle pepper in adobo
- 12 ounces lite lager beer
- 4 cups chicken stock
- 2 cups ketchup
- ¼ cup yellow mustard
- ½ cup apple cider vinegar
- 1 cup firmly packed light brown sugar
- 2 tablespoons Worcestershire sauce
- 2 cups yellow corn kernels (about 2 ears)
- 1 pound tomatoes, grilled and chopped (about 3 cups)
- 3 cups fresh or frozen lima beans, cooked and drained
- 4 cups chopped Beer-Brined Chicken
- 1 teaspoon freshly ground black pepper

Directions:

1. Preheat the grill to 450°F using direct heat with a cast iron grate installed. Preheat the Dutch Oven on the grid for 10 minutes.

2. Place the bacon in the Dutch Oven, close the lid of the grill, and cook until crisp. Using a slotted spoon, transfer the bacon to a small bowl lined with paper towels and set aside. Reserve the bacon fat in the Dutch Oven.

3. Add the barbecue rub to the bacon fat and cook for 1 minute. Add the tomatoes, onions, garlic, and chipotle and cook for 2 to 3 minutes, until the onions are translucent. Slowly add the beer to the Dutch Oven, stirring with a wooden spoon to deglaze. Add the chicken stock, ketchup, mustard, vinegar, brown sugar, and Worcestershire sauce. Leave the Dutch Oven uncovered, but close the lid of the grill. Simmer for 30 minutes, or until the soup has thickened slightly.

4. Remove the Dutch Oven from the heat. Puree the soup using an immersion blender, or carefully spoon it into the bowl of a food processor fitted with the steel blade, process until smooth, and return to the Dutch Oven. Add the corn, grilled tomatoes, lima beans, chicken, and pepper and stir until completely combined. Serve topped with the reserved bacon pieces.

Jamaican Jerk Chicken Wings

Servings:4

Cooking Time: 20 Minutes

Ingredients:

- 6 scallions, greens part only
- 1 tablespoon finely minced fresh ginger
- 1 teaspoon ground allspice
- 1 tablespoon fresh thyme
- 1 tablespoon dark brown sugar
- 1/2 cup fresh orange juice
- 1/4 cup white vinegar
- 1/4 cup soy sauce
- 1/2 cup olive oil

Directions:

1. Preheat the grill to 350°F using direct heat with a cast iron grate installed.
2. Puree all ingredients in a blender until smooth. Pour over chicken wings. Marinate for about 24 hours. Grill wings until done. Serve hot!

Ultimate Chicken Curry

Servings:4

Cooking Time: 27 Minutes

Ingredients:

- 2 tablespoons canola oil
- 1 small onion, coarsely chopped
- 4 pieces of fresh ginger (each about the size and thickness of a 25 cent coin; no need to peel the skin), coarsely chopped
- 2 teaspoons of Raghavan's Blend (page 39 of Indian Cooking Unfolded) or store-bought Madras curry powder
- ½ cup canned diced tomatoes with their juices
- ½ cup half-and-half
- 1 ½ pounds skinless, boneless chicken breasts, cut into 2-inch cubes
- 1 teaspoon coarse kosher or sea salt
- 2 tablespoons finely chopped fresh cilantro leaves and tender stems

Directions:

1. Preheat the grill to 400°F using direct heat with a cast iron grate installed.

2. Heat the oil in a Stir-fry and Paella Pan; once the oil appears to shimmer, add the onion, garlic and ginger and stir-fry until the onion is light caramel brown around the edges (4 to 5 minutes).

3. Sprinkle the spice blend into the pan and stir to mix. Let the spices roast in the onion medley until the aromas dramatically change (10 seconds). Pour in the tomatoes and stir once or twice. By adjusting the upper and lower air vents, begin to lower the heat to 300ºF and simmer the chunky sauce, uncovered, stirring occasionally, until the tomato pieces soften, the excess moisture evaporates, and some of the oils in the spices start to dot the edge of the sauce (5 to 7 minutes).

4. Pour the half-and-half into the pan and scrape the bottom once or twice to release any bits of onion, garlic, and ginger, effectively deglazing the pan and releasing those flavors back into the sauce. Transfer the chunky curry to a blender. Holding the lid down, puree the curry until it is slightly curdled looking but smooth, and saffron orange-hued.

5. Return the sauce to the pan and stir in the chicken and salt. Simmer the curry with the dome closed, stirring occasionally, until the chicken, when cut with a fork or knife, is cooked through, no longer pinkish-red, and its juices run clear (12 to 15 minutes).

6. Sprinkle the cilantro on top of the chicken curry and serve.

Grilled Chicken Arugula Pesto Wings

Servings:4

Cooking Time: 20 Minutes

Ingredients:

- 2 pounds chicken wings, tips trimmed
- 2 teaspoons Better Than Bouillon Seasoned Vegetable Base
- 1 (4 ounce) package of Baby Arugula
- 1 Tablespoon minced garlic
- 1 Tablespoon freshly squeezed lemon juice
- 1/2 teaspoon cracked black pepper
- 3/4 cup grated Parmesan cheese, divided
- 1/2 cup olive oil

Directions:

1. Add the Seasoned Vegetable Base, arugula, garlic, lemon juice, black pepper and 1/4 cup of the Parmesan cheese to the bowl of a food processor fitted with the steel blade. Pulse for 30 seconds. While the machine is running slowly drizzle in the olive oil until the pesto is combined.

2. Add the pesto to a re-sealable plastic bag, add the wings, toss to coat and refrigerate for 2 hours or up to 8 hours.

3. Preheat the grill to 450°F using direct heat with a cast iron grate installed.

4. Remove the wings from the pesto and place directly onto the kamado grill. Grill the wings for 10 minutes per side.

5. Remove the wings from the kamado grill and sprinkle with the remaining grated Parmesan cheese. Serve immediately.

Greek Isles Marinated Chicken

Servings:4

Cooking Time: 60 Minutes

Ingredients:

- ¼ cup water
- 2 BOU Chicken Bouillon Cubes
- 1 tbsp Lemon Pepper Seasoning
- 1 tsp Montreal Steak Seasoning
- ½ cup fresh lemon juice
- 1 tbsp oregano, dry
- ½ cup canola oil
- ¼ cup Italian parsley, chopped
- Zest from 1 lemon
- 1 Roasting Chicken (3½ to 3¾ lbs.)
- 5 oz arugula OR Italian parsley

- 3 tbsp oregano leaves, chopped
- 10 oz grape tomatoes, cut in half
- 2 tsp garlic, minced
- ½ cup red onions, sliced thin
- 4 oz crumbled Greek Feta cheese
- 4 oz Kalamata olives, cut in half
- 5 tbsp olive oil
- 2½ tbsp red wine vinegar
- Salt and black pepper to taste

Directions:

1. Combine all ingredients (except for the chicken) in a blender and blend well.

2. Add the chicken breasts to a stainless steel bowl and coat with the marinade. Marinate for 3 to 4 hours under refrigeration; tossing 2 to 3 times during the marinating time. Or place the chicken into a large 2-gallon resealable bag. Pour the marinade into the bag and seal. Shake to coat the chicken and place under refrigeration (repeat 2 to 3 times during the marinating time).

3. Preheat the grill to 350°F using direct heat with a cast iron grate installed.

4. Remove the chicken from the marinade and allow the excess marinade to drain off. Place the chicken onto a Ceramic Vertical Roaster (fill the roaster with a beer or BOU broth); set the roaster into a Roasting & Drip Pan and place on the cooking grid.

5. Cook to an internal temperature of 165°F in the breast and 175°F in the thigh. Serve with Tomato Feta Salad.

6. Combine all ingredients and toss. Do not over-mix. Place into a serving bowl and serve with Greek Isles Chicken.

Beer Can Chicken

Servings: 6

Cooking Time: 60 Minutes

Ingredients:

- 1 (4-5 lb) chicken
- 1/4 cup Country Style Rub
- 1 (12-ounce) beer in a can
- 1 sprig rosemary
- 2 cloves garlic, smashed

Directions:

1. Open the beer, drink half.
2. Add rosemary and garlic cloves to the remaining beer.
3. Sprinkle Country Style Rub on every surface, inside and out, of the chicken.
4. Situate the chicken on top of the beer can until the can is firmly inside of the cavity.
5. Grilling:
6. Preheat the grill to 375°F using direct heat with a cast iron grate installed.
7. Place the chicken with the beer can standing up on the grid.
8. Close the dome and allow the chicken to cook for 45 minutes to 1 hour or until the internal temperature of the thigh reaches 170°F.
9. Allow the chicken to rest of the heat for 10 minutes before removing the beer can and carving.
10. To cut the spine out of a chicken is called to "spatchcock". This not only allows you to place a brick on top of the bird, but also speeds up the cooking process. Using kitchen shears, cut up one side of the spine and down the other removing it completely. Then, flip the chicken breast side up and press firmly to flatten.

Smoky Grilled Chicken Wings

Servings:6

Cooking Time: 25 Minutes

Ingredients:

- Smoked Paprika Chimichurri
- Marinated Chicken Wings
- ⅔ cup Arugula Leaves, tightly packed
- 1 ⅔ cup Garlic Clove, peeled, finely chopped
- ¼ cup Rosemary Leaves, tightly packed
- 2 cup Italian Parsley Leaves, tightly packed
- ⅔ cup Shallots, finely diced
- 2 tbsp Sage Leaves, tightly packed
- ½ cup Oregano Leaves, tightly packed
- ½ cup Whole Grain Mustard
- 1 ⅔ cup Extra Virgin Olive Oil
- 2 tbsp Smoked Paprika
- 1 tsp Crushed Red Chili Flakes
- ½ cup Red Wine Vinegar
- To taste Sea Salt
- 2 ⅔ cup Water
- ½ cup White Wine Vinegar
- ⅔ cup Lemon Juice
- 2 ½ pounds Chicken Wings
- 1 tbsp Crushed Red Chili Flake
- ¼ cup White Wine Vinegar
- ¾ cup Smoked Paprika Chimichurri
- To taste Fine Sea Salt

Directions:

1. Preheat the grill to 400°F using direct heat with a cast iron grate installed.

2. Place marinated wings on a flat tray and season to taste with sea salt. Place the wings on the kamado grill in a single layer to begin cooking. Allow the skin to begin crisping on one side, then flip and close the lid of the grill to allow the wings to slowly bake as the skin renders crispy. Also closing the lid of the grill will allow the wings to develop that signature smoky flavor that is produced during the cooking process. Maintain a temperature of around 350°F/177°C and check and rotate the wings every 5 minutes to get an even golden brown and crispy skin. The entire process may take anywhere from 20 – 25 minutes. Remove the wings from the heat and place on a wire rack once all the fat is rendered and the skin is evenly crispy and golden brown.

3. Allow to rest for 3 – 5 minutes, then serve.

4. Finely chop all herbs and greens. Combine all finely chopped herbs in a large mixing bowl. Add remainder of the ingredients and mix thoroughly. Reserve finished chimichurri in the refrigerator until ready for use.

5. On a clean cutting board with a sharp knife separate the drumette, flap, and wing tip; discard the wing tips. In a large bowl combine the vinegar, chimichurri, and red chili flakes. Toss the drumettes and flaps in the chimichurri marinade until well coated and allow to sit in the refrigerator for 3½ – 4 hours.

Cuban Chicken Bombs

Servings: 4

Cooking Time: 30 Minutes

Ingredients:

- 4 bone in chicken thighs
- 4 slices of ham (cut into quarters)
- 4 slices of provolone (cut into quarters)
- 2 tbsp Dijon mustard
- 12 pickle chips
- 8 slices of bacon
- Sweet & Smoky Seasoning

Directions:

1. Preheat the grill to 300°F using direct heat with a cast iron grate installed.

2. Debone the chicken thighs leaving the skin on and position the chicken thighs skin side down. Spread equal portions of the mustard on the meat side of each chicken thigh. Place an equal amount of provolone slices, ham and pickles on each chicken thigh. Roll the chicken thighs up and wrap a piece of bacon around the middle of the chicken thigh and another around the thigh lengthwise sealing the contents with bacon. Put toothpicks through the bottom of the chicken thighs to help keep contents inside while cooking. Season the top of the bacon with the Sweet & Smokey Seasoning.

3. Cook the chicken for about an hour or until the internal temperature reaches 165°F. Remove the chicken from the kamado grill and let rest before slicing and serving.

Walk The Plank Chicken Quarters

Servings: 4

Cooking Time: 60 Minutes

Ingredients:

- 4 chicken leg quarters (drumstick and thigh)
- 4 cups Maple Brine
- 1/4 cup Coffee Spice Barbecue Sauce
- 2 untreated cedar planks

Directions:

1. In a large zip top bag, pour cool Maple Brine over chicken leg quarters and allow them to sit, refrigerated, for 2 hours.

2. Remove the chicken from the brine, pat dry, and allow to come to room temperature while the grill is heating.

3. Grilling:

4. Preheat the grill to 350°F using direct heat with a cast iron grate installed. Place the cedar planks on the grid for 3 minutes, with the dome closed.

5. Flip the plank and place the chicken on the heated side. Close the dome for 45 minutes to 1 hour or until the thigh registers 170°F.

6. Generously brush the thighs with Coffee Spice Barbecue Sauce and close the dome for an additional 5 minutes. Serve with additional sauce.

BEEF

Surf And Turf Rolls

Servings:8
Cooking Time: 60 Minutes

Ingredients:

- 1 lb (450 g) beef tenderloin
- 8 shrimp or prawns (size 8/12 count)
- 1 clove of garlic, peeled and finely chopped
- Olive oil
- 2 1/2 cups (40 g) rocket (arugula)
- 3 oz (85 g) dried tomatoes
- 7 oz (200 g) pig caul, thoroughly washed*
- Lime juice
- 4 Cobs in Husks
- Butter
- Finely shredded zest of 1/2 lemon
- 2 egg yolks
- 2 tbsp (30 ml) wholegrain mustard
- 1 dash white balsamic vinegar
- 3.5 oz (100 ml) vegetable oil
- 1.75 oz (50 ml) olive oil
- 1 passion fruit
- 1 tablespoon sour cream
- Juice of 1/2 lemon

Directions:

1. Preheat the grill to 210°F using direct heat with a cast iron grate installed.
2. Cut the beef tenderloin into four equal portions. Wrap each piece of meat in plastic wrap and flatten with the underside of a frying pan.
3. Peel the prawns, remove the intestine and rinse with water. In a bowl, coat the prawns with some olive oil, plus the garlic and salt and pepper to taste. Wash the rocket and slice the tomatoes.
4. Remove the meat from the wrap and distribute the rocket and tomato slices over the meat. Place 2 prawns in the center of each piece of meat, roll up tightly and wrap in a piece of pork caul or secure with toothpicks. Put the rolls on the cooking grid, close the lid and cook for 20 minutes.
5. Remove the rolls from the grid and cover with foil. Using a Pit Mitt or barbecue mitt, carefully add the platesetter and replace the Cast Iron Grid; heat the kamado grill to 350°F.
6. Take the cobs and the rolls off the grill. Remove the husk and silk and spread the cobs immediately with butter.
7. Cut the rolls into slices and drizzle with lime juice. Divide across the plates and serve with the mayonnaise and a delicious rocket salad.
8. Keeping the husks intact, snip the silks from the top of the corn and moisten the cobs in water. Place the cobs on the grid and grill for about 35 minutes, turning regularly until the husk has blackened evenly. For the final 5 minutes of the preparation time add the rolls and cook until nice and brown.
9. Prepare the mayonnaise by blending together the egg yolks, mustard, lemon zest and balsamic vinegar. Stirring all the time, pour in the vegetable oil and olive oil, one drop at a time and then in a small trickle, to create a creamy mayonnaise. Cut the passion fruit in half, scoop out the flesh and mix with the sour cream. Add to the mayonnaise along with the lemon juice and salt and pepper to taste.

Smoked Beef Tenderloin

Servings: 8

Cooking Time: 120 Minutes

Ingredients:

- 1 whole beef tenderloin, about 5lb (2.3kg) in total, trimmed
- 1/4 cup extra virgin olive oil
- kosher salt and freshly ground black pepper
- 4 garlic cloves, minced
- 1/4 cup chopped fresh basil
- 1/4 cup chopped fresh rosemary
- 1/4 cup chopped fresh oregano
- 1/4 cup chopped fresh marjoram
- 1/4 cup chopped fresh flat-leaf parsley
- 8 hoagie rolls, to serve
- for the sauce
- 2 tbsp mustard seeds
- 1/4 cup Dijon mustard
- 1/4 cup whole grain mustard
- 5 tbsp mayonnaise
- 5 tbsp sour cream
- 21/4 tsp Worcestershire sauce
- to smoke
- alder, hickory, or apricot wood chunks

Directions:

1. Rub beef with oil, salt, pepper, garlic, basil, rosemary, oregano, marjoram, and parsley. Wrap tightly with plastic wrap and refrigerate for 4 to 24 hours.

2. To make the sauce, in a medium bowl, combine mustard seeds, Dijon mustard, whole grain mustard, mayonnaise, sour cream, and Worcestershire sauce. Cover the bowl and refrigerate for 1 hour or overnight to allow the flavors to meld.

3. Preheat the grill to 225°F (107°C). Once hot, add the wood chunks and install the heat deflector and a standard grate. Place tenderloin on the grate, close the lid, and smoke until the internal temperature reaches 125°F (52°C), about 1 to 2 hours.

4. Transfer beef to a cutting board and let rest for 15 minutes. While the meat rests, place rolls on the grate cut side down and lightly toast, about 2 to 3 minutes. Thinly slice the meat. To serve, spread the mustard cream sauce on the rolls and pile on the beef.

Italian Meatballs

Servings: 12

Cooking Time: 30 Minutes

Ingredients:

- 1/4 cup panko breadcrumbs, lightly toasted
- 3/4lb (340g) Roma tomatoes, peeled and chopped
- 2 tbsp extra virgin olive oil, divided
- 1/2 tbsp nonpareil capers, drained and chopped
- 1/2 tsp dried oregano
- 1/2 tsp dried marjoram
- 1 tbsp fresh basil, plus more for serving, chopped
- 1/3lb (150g) ground pork
- 1/3lb (150g) ground beef
- 1/3lb (150g) ground veal
- 3 tsp whole milk
- 1 large egg, lightly beaten
- 2 pitted Kalamata olives, minced
- 1 tbsp grated Parmesan cheese, plus more for serving
- 1 tbsp fresh flat-leaf parsley, minced
- 1 tsp kosher salt, plus more as needed
- freshly ground black pepper

Directions:

1. Preheat the grill to 375°F (191°C) using indirect heat with a standard grate and a cast iron skillet installed.

2. On a rimmed sheet pan, place breadcrumbs in a single layer and toast until beginning to brown, about 3 to 5 minutes. Remove the pan from the grill and set aside.

3. Place tomatoes in a food processor and purée. Place tomatoes and 1 tbsp oil in the skillet. Bring to a boil, slightly close the top and bottom vents to reduce the temperature to 325°F (163°C), close the lid, and simmer until the sauce starts to thicken, about 5 minutes, stirring occasionally.

4. Add capers, oregano, and marjoram to the skillet, and simmer until the sauce has reduced to 11/4 cups, about 5 minutes. Add basil, season with salt to taste, and set aside.

5. In a large bowl, combine pork, beef, and veal. Add breadcrumbs, milk, egg, olives, Parmesan cheese, parsley, and salt, and mix well with your hands. Shape the mixture into 12 meatballs.

6. Slightly open the top and bottom vents to return the temperature to 375°F (191°C). Once the grill reaches the needed temperature, return the skillet to the grill and heat the remaining 1 tbsp oil until shimmering. Place the meatballs in the skillet, close the lid, and cook until they start to brown, about 8 minutes, turning once every 2 minutes. Add the sauce, close the lid, and cook until the meatballs are cooked through and the sauce is hot, about 8 minutes.

7. Remove the meatballs from the grill, place on a large serving platter, and top with more Parmesan cheese and basil. Serve immediately.

Smoked Canuck Chili

Servings: 10
Cooking Time: 180 Minutes

Ingredients:

- 2lb (1kg) lean ground beef
- 1/2 large yellow onion, diced
- 3 tbsp garlic powder
- 1 tbsp seasoned pepper
- 2 tbsp crushed red pepper flakes, plus more to taste
- 2 x 4oz (133g) cans mushroom pieces, drained
- 28oz (794g) can baked beans
- 2 x 15oz (425g) cans kidney beans, with liquid
- 2 x 6oz (150g) cans tomato paste
- 1/4 cup sugar
- 3 medium carrots, diced
- 3 celery stalks, diced
- 1 red bell pepper, diced
- 2 jalapeño peppers, diced
- 1/4 cup lager beer
- 1/4 cup BBQ sauce
- 2 tsp hot sauce, plus more to taste
- to smoke
- maple or alder wood chunks

Directions:

1. Preheat the grill to 325°F (163°C) using indirect heat with a dutch oven on the heat deflector. To the hot dutch oven, add beef, onion, garlic powder, seasoned pepper, and red pepper flakes. Close the lid and cook until the meat has browned, about 5 to 10 minutes. Remove the dutch oven and heat deflector, drain off the fat, and add wood chunks to the coals.

2. Reinstall the heat deflector and replace the dutch oven. Add mushrooms, baked beans, kidney beans with liquid, tomato paste, sugar, carrots, celery, pepper, jalapeños, beer, BBQ sauce, and hot sauce to the dutch oven. Stir to combine, and season with more red pepper flakes and hot sauce to taste.

3. Close the top and bottom vents most of the way to lower the grill temperature to 225°F (107°C). Leaving the dutch oven uncovered, close the grill lid, and smoke for 2 to 3 hours.

4. Remove the dutch oven from the grill, and serve immediately.

Moroccan Meatball Sliders

Servings:8

Cooking Time: 16 Minutes

Ingredients:

- 1 pound ground beef
- 3⁄4 cup panko bread crumbs
- 3⁄4 cup diced onions
- 1⁄2 cup Sabra Classic Hummus
- 21⁄2 tablespoons tandoori spice blend (such as Spiceologist Tandoori Glory, see notes) 2 tablespoons minced cilantro
- 1 egg, lightly beaten
- 1 teaspoon kosher salt
- 1 teaspoon ground pepper
- 8 mini bagels
- Sabra Greek Yogurt Onion Dip (or other onion dip)

Directions:

1. Preheat the grill to 400°F using direct heat with a cast iron grate installed.

2. In a medium bowl add the ingredients – ground beef through ground pepper – and mix just until combined. Use a large hinged scoop or a spoon and make meatballs about 2 1⁄2 inches in circumference. Place on a parchment lined plate and continue with remaining meat mixture.

3. Add the meatballs to the cooking grid and cook for about 15 minutes or until no longer pink inside, turning every few minutes to cook on each side. Toast the bagel halves for 1 minute on grill. Remove and assemble by placing a meatball on 8 of the bagel halves, spread a tablespoon of Greek yogurt dip on the bagel top and press onto the meatballs. Use a toothpick to hold them in place (optional). Serve immediately.

Smoked Beef Brisket

Servings: 38
Cooking Time: 900 Minutes

Ingredients:

- 1 1/4 cups sugar
- 2/3 cup ground black pepper
- 2/3 cup seasoned salt
- 2/3 cup kosher salt
- 2 1/2 tbsp ground cayenne pepper
- 15lb (6.8kg) whole beef brisket, trimmed of fat
- pickle slices (optional), to serve
- BBQ sauce (optional), to serve
- to smoke
- post oak, hickory, or mesquite wood chunks

Directions:

1. In a medium bowl, combine sugar, pepper, seasoned salt, kosher salt, and cayenne. Rub brisket with the seasoning mixture. Wrap tightly with plastic wrap and refrigerate for 24 hours.
2. Preheat the grill to 225°F (107°C). Once hot, add the wood chunks, install the heat deflector, place a drip pan on top, and install a standard grate. Remove brisket from the fridge and allow to come to room temperature.
3. Place the brisket fat side up on the grate, close the lid, and smoke until the internal temperature reaches 160°F (71°C), about 5 to 7 hours. Remove brisket from the grill, wrap heavily in aluminum foil, and return to the grill to continue to cook until the internal temperature reaches 185°F (85°C), about 8 hours. (Check the texture of the meat for doneness throughout the cooking process). The total cook time is about 15 hours, or 1 hour per pound (approximately 2 hours per kilogram).
4. Transfer brisket to a serving platter and let rest for 20 minutes. Slice or shred the meat, and serve with pickle slices and BBQ sauce (if desired).

Corned Beef And Cabbage

Servings:8
Cooking Time: 30 Minutes

Ingredients:

- 3 pounds corned beef brisket with spice packet
- 1 can or bottle Irish Stout
- 10 small red potatoes
- 5 carrots, peeled and cut into 3-inch pieces
- 1 large head cabbage, cut into large wedges
- 2 bay leaves

Directions:

1. Preheat the grill to 450°F using direct heat with a cast iron grate installed.
2. Place the corned beef in the dutch oven and cover with water and the stout; add the spice packet that came with the corned beef and cover. Place on the cooking grid and bring to a boil, then reduce the temperature to 350°F. Simmer approximately 50 minutes per pound or until tender.
3. After two hours, add whole potatoes and carrots, and cook for 15 minutes. Add cabbage and cook for 15 more minutes. Remove meat and let rest for 15 minutes.
4. Place vegetables in a bowl and cover with some of the broth. Slice meat across the grain and serve with warm bread.

Smash Cheese Burgers

Servings:4

Cooking Time: 5 Minutes

Ingredients:

- 1 lb ground beef
- 1 tbsp garlic powder
- Salt and pepper to taste
- 8 slices of cheddar cheese, optional

Directions:

1. Preheat the grill to 500°F using direct heat with a cast iron grate installed.
2. Season the beef with garlic powder, salt and pepper. Roll beef into 8 – 2 oz. balls.
3. Place 4 balls on the plancha, close the lid and wait 1-2 minutes. Open the lid and smash the balls with a spatula until they are about an inch thick. Cook 2 minutes. Flip the burgers and cook another 2 minutes. Put cheese on the burger and wait another minute, until the cheese is melted. Repeat with the remaining balls.
4. Top with your favorite toppings.

Frankie Ballard's Rib-eye Steaks

Servings:6

Cooking Time: 10 Minutes

Ingredients:

- 4 bone-in rib-eyes
- Salt and pepper
- 1 tablespoon unsalted butter
- ¼ cup mushrooms, cut to bite size
- ¼ cup chopped leeks
- 1 clove garlic, minced
- ½ cup whiskey
- 2 cups heavy cream
- ⅛ tsp cayenne pepper
- Salt and pepper

Directions:

1. Preheat the grill to 650°F using direct heat with a cast iron grate installed.
2. Coat both sides of the steak with salt and lots of pepper.
3. Set a cast iron skillet or dutch oven on the grid and let it heat up for a few minutes. Add the butter and cook it until it is slightly brown, then add the mushrooms and cook until tender. Stir in the leeks and garlic.
4. Put the steaks on the grid and close the lid. Grill for about 4 minutes for medium-rare, turning once. Move the steaks to plates. Pour the sauce over the steaks and serve – they won't last long!
5. Slowly add the whiskey; it will ignite, so seriously, add it slowly! Once the whiskey burns off, stir and close the lid of the grill. Cook until the whiskey reduces by two-thirds. Add the cream, and stir frequently for 3 to 4 minutes. The sauce will thicken up and will coat a wooden spoon, that's when you know it's ready! Add a little cayenne pepper and then add salt and pepper if you'd like.

Homemade Pastrami

Servings: 16
Cooking Time: 720 Minutes

Ingredients:

- 15lb (6.8kg) beef brisket
- for the brine
- 1 cup kosher salt
- 1 gallon (3.8 liters) water
- 2 tsp ground coriander
- 1 cup packed dark brown sugar
- 2 tsp pink curing salt
- 1 tsp ground juniper berries
- 1/2 tsp ground ginger
- 1/2 tsp granulated garlic
- 1/2 tsp ground cloves
- for the rub
- 1/2 cup coarse ground black pepper
- 1/4 cup ground coriander
- 2 tsp mustard powder
- 2 tbsp light brown sugar
- 2 tbsp paprika
- 4 tsp garlic powder
- 4 tsp onion powder
- to smoke
- hickory, oak, or apple, wood chunks

Directions:

1. In a stockpot or other large vessel, combine all the brine ingredients and bring to a boil on the stovetop over high heat. Remove the vessel from the heat and refrigerate to allow to cool completely. (Any extra brine can be refrigerated and saved for a later use.) Once the brine has cooled, submerge brisket in the brine, cover with plastic wrap, and refrigerate for 5 to 8 days.

2. Remove brisket from the curing liquid and pat dry with paper towels. In a small bowl, combine all the rub ingredients. Thoroughly coat brisket on all sides with the rub. Wrap tightly in plastic wrap and refrigerate for 24 hours.

3. Preheat the grill to 225°F (107°C). Once hot, add the wood chunks and install the heat deflector and a standard grate. Place brisket on the grate and smoke until the internal temperature reaches 185°F (85°C), about 12 hours.

4. Remove brisket from the grill and let rest for 30 minutes before slicing and serving.

Smoked Brisket Roll

Servings:10

Cooking Time: 650 Minutes

Ingredients:

- 1 brisket flat, fat cap on, about 6 lbs (2.7 kg)
- 1 cup brisket rub
- ½ bag Jack Daniels wood chips, soaked overnight in water
- Bardough House Slaw
- 10 country loaf rolls
- Salted farm butter for the rolls
- 1½ cups (360 ml) brown sugar
- 1 cup (240 ml) kosher salt
- 1 cup (240 ml) ground espresso beans
- ¼ cup (60 ml) freshly ground black pepper
- ¼ cup (60 ml) garlic powder
- 2 Tbsp (30 ml) ground cinnamon
- 2 Tbsp (30 ml) ground cumin
- 2 Tbsp (30 ml) cayenne pepper
- 1½ cups (150 g) green cabbage, thinly sliced
- 1½ cups (150 g) red cabbage, thinly sliced
- 1¼ cups (150 g) julienned carrots
- 1/3 cup (40 g) dried cranberries
- 2 Tbsp (30 ml) mustard
- 1 cup (240 ml) mayo
- Salt to taste
- 1 lb (455 g) stone ground flour
- 1½ cups (355 g) filtered water
- 2¼ tsp (7 g) fresh yeast
- 5 g salt
- 3 Tbsp + 1 tsp (50 ml) extra virgin olive oil

Directions:

1. Coat the brisket on all sides with an even layer of rub. Let the meat to rest for 1 hour at room temperature or until the rub starts to turn pasty.

2. Preheat the grill to 225°F using direct heat with a cast iron grate installed.

3. Place the brisket, fat side up, on the grill. After 8 hours check meat periodically. Poke the meat in a few places; the fat should separate under your finger. When the brisket reaches an internal temperature of 200°F, remove it from the kamado grill onto a rimmed baking sheet to rest for 30 minutes.

4. Cut the brisket in thin slices against the grain. Cut the rolls in half and butter on both sides. Add sliced brisket and slaw and enjoy!

5. Mix all rub ingredients together and refrigerate.

6. Mix all slaw ingredients together and refrigerate.

7. Dissolve the yeast in half the water. Place the flour and salt in a mixing bowl; add the yeast mixture and the oil.

8. Knead the dough by hand for 10 minutes, slowly adding the rest of the water. Allow to rest for 1 hour or until double in size. Divide into 10 equal size rounds. Shape into balls and allow to rest for an additional hour.

9. Set the kamado grill for indirect cooking with the platesetter and a Pizza and Baking Stone at 400°F. Place the rolls 1 inch (2.5 cm) apart on the preheated stone. Spritz lightly with water and bake for 15 minutes, then remove to a cooling rack.

Grilled Italian Meatloaf Sandwich

Servings: 4

Cooking Time: 140 Minutes

Ingredients:

- 2 pounds of 80% lean ground beef
- ½ cup shredded Parmesan cheese
- 1 tablespoon Worcestershire sauce
- ¼ cup of marinara sauce (save extra from the jar for brushing on top of the meatloaf)
- 1 cup of breadcrumbs
- ½ teaspoon black pepper
- ¾ teaspoon kosher salt
- 3 eggs
- 2 teaspoon red pepper flakes
- 2 tablespoons dried parsley
- 2 tablespoons dried basil
- 2 tablespoons dried oregano
- ½ cup of diced sweet onion
- 1 tablespoon of diced garlic
- ½ cup of minced carrots
- Cobblestone Bread Co (TM) Toasted Onions Rolls
- Sliced Mozzarella Cheese

Directions:

1. Lightly mix the ingredients together in a large bowl. Form the meatloaf on a grilling plank and let it rest a few minutes.

2. Preheat the grill to 350°F using direct heat with a cast iron grate installed. Cook for approximately 2 hours. With one hour left, take additional marinara sauce and brush it on top of the meatloaf. Repeat every 15-20 minutes until a nice tomato glaze has formed on top. The meatloaf is cooked when the meat registers 165°F in the center.

3. Let the meatloaf rest and cool a bit. Take the Cobblestone Bread Co (TM) Toasted Onion Rolls and lightly grill them for about 30 seconds to get warm. Slice the meatloaf thick and assemble the sandwich by placing the meatloaf on the roll and topping it with a slice of mozzarella cheese.

Dr. Bbq's Roasted Upside Down Chili

Servings:6

Cooking Time: 120 Minutes

Ingredients:

- ¼ cup olive oil
- 1 large yellow onion, chopped
- 1 large green pepper, seeded and chopped
- 2 jalapenos, finely chopped
- 4 cloves garlic, crushed
- 1 28-oz can diced tomatoes
- 1 quart beef broth
- 1 cup Vidalia Onion Sriracha Barbecue Sauce
- ⅓ cup chili powder
- 2 tbsp ground cumin
- 1 tbsp brown sugar
- 1 tsp cayenne pepper
- 3 lbs coarse ground beef, formed into a large patty
- 2 15-oz can of dark kidney beans, drained

Directions:

1. Preheat the grill to 350°F using direct heat with a cast iron grate installed.

2. Add a dutch oven (uncovered) to the grid. Add the oil, then add the onion and green pepper and cook until soft. Add the garlic and jalapenos and cook a few more minutes. Add the tomatoes, broth, barbecue sauce, chili powder, cumin, brown sugar and pepper. Mix well and bring to a simmer.

3. Remove the dutch oven and the cooking grid, and then add a couple small chunks of apple wood. Add an grillspander with a platesetter for indirect tiered cooking. Place the dutch oven on the bottom grid and continue cooking.

4. Season the ground beef patty with salt and pepper, and then place the ground beef patty on the top sliding grid, centered over the dutch oven so that the meat drips into the chili. Cook for 1½ hours, adjusting the heat to maintain a simmer.

5. Remove the meat to a sheet pan. Add the beans to the chili and add more water if needed. Break the meat up with tongs and place it in the pot. Cook for another 30 minutes until everything is well blended and slightly thickened.

Taco Soup

Servings: 8
Cooking Time: 60 Minutes

Ingredients:

- 1 lb ground beef
- 4 cups chicken broth
- 1/2 cup chopped onion
- 1 Tablespoon garlic, minced
- 1 Tablespoon chili powder
- 1 Tablespoon smoked paprika
- 1 tsp ground cumin
- 2 cans pinto beans, rinsed and drained
- 1 can black beans, rinsed and drained
- 1 can corn, drained
- Salt & Pepper

Directions:

1. Place ingredients in a cold dutch oven and stir.
2. Grilling:
3. Preheat the grill to 350°F using direct heat with a cast iron grate installed.
4. Place the dutch oven on the grid of the grill and lower the dome for 1 hour.
5. Soup is done when the ground beef is cooked through.
6. Serve with shredded cheese, cut up avocado, shredded cabbage and tortilla chips.

Italian Sausage Sliders

Servings:16
Cooking Time: 6 Minutes

Ingredients:

- 2 pounds Johnsonville All Natural Ground Italian Sausage or Links (remove from casing)
- 1 pound ground beef
- 16 small slider buns or mini sandwich rolls
- Condiments
- Provolone cheese and Marinara sauce
- Fresh mozzarella, fresh basil, and sliced tomatoes
- Giardiniera – marinated chopped vegetables and olives
- Sauteed onions and roasted red peppers
- Sauteed mushrooms and Cheddar cheese

Directions:

1. Preheat the grill to 400°F using direct heat with a cast iron grate installed.
2. In a large bowl, combine sausage and beef. Using your hands, blend the two meats together and form into one large ball. Use a spoon or a small measuring cup to gather up about a 3 ounce ball and press into patties … with the Mini Burger Basket you can form and cook 12 Mini Burgers at once!
3. Place the Mini Burger Basket or individual sliders directly on the cooking grid. Cook for about 3 minutes then flip and continue cooking for another 3 minutes. The internal temperature should be 160°F.
4. Slice the buns and top the sliders with your favorite condiments.

Grilled Top Blade Steak

Servings:4

Cooking Time: 7 Minutes

Ingredients:

- 2 top-blade steaks (about 1½ pounds), 1 to 1¼-inches thick Kosher salt
- 2 thick slices artisan bread, crusts removed and torn into ragged 1½-inch pieces
- 2 tablespoons extra-virgin olive oil, divided
- 1 teaspoon sherry or red wine vinegar
- 5 ounces baby arugula (about 6 cups)
- 1 cup lightly packed fresh herb leaves, such as basil, parsley, dill, chives, chervil, tarragon, mint, or a combination
- Finishing salt, such as coarse sea salt or flake salt
- Freshly ground black pepper

Directions:

1. Pat the steaks dry with a paper towel and season liberally with the kosher salt. Toss the bread with 1 tablespoon of the olive oil and set it aside.

2. Preheat the grill to 450°F using direct heat with a cast iron grate installed, scrape the grid clean, and oil it lightly. Cook the steaks on the hottest part of the grill until seared, 3 to 3½ minutes. Use tongs to flip them and sear the second side for another 3 to 3½ minutes for medium rare. (To cook the steaks medium or beyond, slide them over to the coolest part of the kamado grill and close the cover, then cook for 1 to 4 minutes more.)

3. Grill the reserved bread croutons while the steaks rest, turning them 2 to 3 times, until they are tinged with brown.

4. Transfer the steaks to a cutting board. While they rest, make the salad dressing by whisking the vinegar with the remaining 1 tablespoon olive oil in a small bowl. Put the arugula and herbs in a salad bowl and toss with the dressing. Slice the steak against the grain into ½-inch-thick slices and put 4 to 5 slices on each plate. Pile a portion of the salad on top of each serving and balance a few croutons on top. Drizzle any meat juices from the cutting board over it all and sprinkle to taste with the finishing salt and black pepper.

The Perfect Steak

Servings:2

Cooking Time: 5 Minutes

Ingredients:
- 2 steaks, 1-1/2 to 2-inches thick, preferably ribeye or strip
- Ancho Chile & Coffee Seasoning, to taste

Directions:
1. Trim the steaks of any excess fat. Apply the seasoning to both sides of the steaks. Allow to stand at room temperature for 30 minutes before grilling.
2. Preheat the grill to 650°F using direct heat with a cast iron grate installed. To increase sear marks use a cast iron cooking grid; for extra flavor add wood chips.
3. Place the steaks on the grill and sear for two to three minutes. Carefully open the dome and flip the steaks onto a new section of the grid. After two to three more minutes, flip the steaks once more.
4. Completely shut down the kamado grill by closing the damper top and draft door. Let the steaks continue cooking for 3 to 4 minutes, until they reach the desired internal temperature (check with a meat thermometer).
5. Remove the steaks and let them rest for 5 minutes before serving.

Pitmaster Ribeyes

Servings: 4

Cooking Time: 75 Minutes

Ingredients:
- 4 ribeye steaks
- 1/4 cup spice rub

Directions:
1. Season both sides of all steaks with spice rub and allow to sit for 15 minutes.
2. Grilling:
3. Preheat the grill to 225°F using direct heat with a cast iron grate installed. Add soaked wood chips to the charcoal. (We like pecan or apple.)
4. Place the steaks on the grid and allow to smoke for 1 hour.
5. Remove the steaks from the grill.
6. Heat the grill to 500°F.
7. Place steaks on the grid and close the dome for 3 minutes.
8. Flip the steaks over and cook an additional 2 minutes.
9. Close all of the vents and let the steaks sit for 5 minutes or until the internal temperature reaches 130°F.
10. Allow the steaks to rest for 5-10 minutes before slicing.

Ancho Chili Steak Tacos

Servings: 2
Cooking Time: 4 Minutes

Ingredients:

- Flank steak
- Ancho Chile & Coffee Seasoning
- Cayenne Hot Sauces
- 1 large red onion
- 4 jalapeno peppers
- Soft flour tortillas (small)

Directions:

1. Preheat the grill to 400°F using direct heat with a cast iron grate installed.
2. Cut the onion in half and grill with the jalapeno until desired doneness.
3. Season the steak with the Ancho Chile & Coffee Seasoning. Grill the flank steak for 2 minutes per side; rest for 2 minutes and then slice thin.
4. Warm the tortillas on the top sliding grid. On each tortilla, add meat and top with the onions. Serve the tacos with sauce on the side.

Braised Short Ribs

Servings: 8
Cooking Time: 130 Minutes

Ingredients:

- 8 bone-in beef short ribs
- 1 tsp salt
- 2 tsp freshly ground black pepper
- 4 tbsp olive oil
- ½ cup yellow onion, diced
- 3 cloves garlic, minced
- 1 cup beef broth
- 3 tbsp Worcestershire sauce
- 1 cup red wine
- 2 sprigs of rosemary

Directions:

1. Preheat the grill to 350°F using direct heat with a cast iron grate installed.
2. Season the short ribs with salt and pepper. Heat olive oil in the dutch oven. Sear short ribs for 1 minute per side. Remove from the dutch oven and set aside.
3. Add the onion to the dutch oven and cook for 3 minutes or until it is translucent. Add in garlic and cook for an additional minute.
4. Pour beef broth, Worcestershire sauce and red wine into the dutch oven. Bring to a simmer and add in the short ribs. Place the rosemary sprigs on top. Cover the dutch oven and cook for 2½ hours, or until meat is tender.

Bacon-wrapped Steakhouse Filet

Servings:2

Cooking Time: 12 Minutes

Ingredients:

- 2 bacon slices
- 2-2½ inch thick filet steaks
- Classic Steakhouse Seasoning
- Extra virgin olive oil
- Skewers

Directions:

1. Preheat the grill to 550°F using direct heat with a cast iron grate installed.
2. On a perforated cooking grid, cook the bacon just until it has firmed up a little bit. Set aside.
3. Coat the steaks with olive oil and season with Classic Steakhouse Seasoning on all sides. Wrap the partially-cooked bacon around the edges of the steak; secure with a skewer.
4. Grill the steaks for 5-6 minutes on each side, or until the internal temperature is 125°F(or to slightly below your desired temperature). Remove from grill and let rest covered for 10 minutes.
5. Slice and serve!

Reverse Sear Tri Tip With Chimichurri

Servings:4

Cooking Time: 10 Minutes

Ingredients:

- 1 - 2 pound, 2-inch-thick tri tip steak
- A coarse seasoning/dry rub with a generous amount of pepper
- Olive oil
- 1½ cup parsley
- 1 cup chopped cilantro
- 1/3 cup oregano
- ¼ cup minced red onion
- 3 tsp. minced garlic
- ½ tbsp. salt
- Juice from 1 lime
- 1 tbsp. white wine vinegar
- 1 cup extra virgin olive oil

Directions:

1. Preheat the grill to 250°F using direct heat with a cast iron grate installed.
2. Rub the tri tip with olive oil and apply a generous amount of seasoning on both sides. Let it rest for about 30 minutes while your kamado grill comes up to temperature.
3. Place the tri tip on the kamado grill and cook until it reaches an internal temperature of 115°F. Remove and cover with foil to let it rest for about 10 minutes.
4. Remove the platesetter and switch to direct heat, and get the kamado grill up to 500°F.Sear the tri tip on high heat for 2-3 minutes per side.
5. Remove and let rest for another 10 minutes. Slice against the grain, and serve with chimichurri.
6. Crush the garlic and salt together to make a paste. Add cilantro, oregano, parsley and red onion and lime juice. Mix ingredients together. Add white wine vinegar and extra virgin olive oil and salt/pepper to taste. Mix thoroughly for even flavor. Use immediately or let rest in the refrigerator overnight for more fuller flavor.

Pulled Beef Sandwich

Servings: 6
Cooking Time: 180 Minutes

Ingredients:

- 3lb (1.4kg) boneless chuck roast
- for the rub
- 1/4 cup packed light brown sugar
- 3 tbsp kosher salt
- 3 tbsp ground black pepper
- 2 tbsp garlic powder
- for the sauce
- 1/4 cup BBQ sauce
- 2 cups ketchup
- 2 tbsp gochujang
- 3 tbsp Worcestershire sauce
- 3 tbsp Dijon mustard
- 1 tbsp kosher salt
- 1/4 tbsp ground black pepper
- to serve
- 6 sandwich buns, split
- sliced onions
- dill pickles
- pickled hot peppers
- to smoke
- hickory wood chunks

Directions:

1. To make the rub, in a small bowl, combine sugar, salt, pepper, and garlic powder. Evenly coat roast with the rub, wrap tightly with plastic wrap, and refrigerate for 24 hours. Remove roast from the fridge and allow to come to room temperature.

2. Preheat the grill to 275°F (135°C). Once hot, add the wood chunks and install the heat deflector and a standard grate. Place roast on the grate, close the lid, and smoke until the internal temperature reaches 165°F (74°C), about 60 to 90 minutes.

3. To make the sauce, in a small bowl, combine BBQ sauce, ketchup, gochujang, Worcestershire sauce, mustard, salt, and pepper. Shape some aluminum foil into a bowl, remove roast from the grill, and place roast in the foil bowl. Coat roast with the sauce, allowing the excess to pool in the foil, and wrap roast tightly to prevent sauce or steam from escaping.

4. Return foil-wrapped roast to the grill, close the lid, and smoke until the internal temperature reaches 185°F (85°C) and the meat shreds easily, about 60 to 90 minutes. Transfer the roast to a large serving platter and let rest 30 minutes, keeping it wrapped in the foil.

5. Unwrap roast, shred with two forks, and pour the sauce from the foil over top. Serve immediately on buns, topping with onions, pickles, and hot peppers or other desired toppings.

Rouladen

Servings: 6
Cooking Time: 45 Minutes

Ingredients:
- 1 (1 1/2-2lb) flank steak
- 1/2 cup chopped onion
- 1/3 cup chopped dill pickle
- 1/4 cup German mustard
- 1/2 tsp salt
- 1/4 tsp pepper
- 6 strips of bacon, separated

Directions:
1. In a medium skillet, brown 3 strips of bacon until crisp. Remove from the pan.
2. Remove all by 2 Tablespoon of the bacon fat and cook the onion over medium heat or until the onion is translucent. Set aside to cool.
3. Pound flank steak into an 8 inch by 10 inch rectangle.
4. Spread the meat with the mustard.
5. Top the meat with the onion, dill pickle, and crumbled cooked bacon.
6. Roll the meat around the filling lengthwise.
7. Wrap the roast with the remaining raw bacon and secure with metal skewers.
8. Grilling:
9. Preheat the grill to 425°F using direct heat with a cast iron grate installed. Place the roast on the grid and cook for 30-45 minutes or until the internal temperature reaches 130°F.
10. Allow the rouladen to rest for 20 minutes before carving.

BURGERS

Breakfast Burger

Servings: 4

Cooking Time: 13 Minutes

Ingredients:

- 1 1/2 lb ground beef
- 1/2 lb ground pork breakfast sausage
- 2 Tablespoon butter
- 8 strips bacon
- 4 slices sharp cheddar cheese
- 4 Brioche buns
- 4 eggs
- 4 thick slices tomato

Directions:

1. In a medium bowl, mix ground beef and sausage until just combined.
2. Form into 4 patties and refrigerate while the grill heats.
3. Melt butter in a large skillet and fry the eggs for 2 minutes on each side.
4. Grilling:
5. Preheat the grill to 400°F using direct heat with a cast iron grate installed.
6. Place bacon on a small cookie sheet and place on the grid in the grill. Cook until crispy.
7. Place the patties on the grid and close the dome for 3 minutes.
8. Flip the burgers and replace the dome for an additional 3 minutes.
9. Close all of the vents and allow the burgers to sit for an additional 5 minutes. The internal temperature of the burger should be 150°F.
10. Place cheese on top of the burgers and cover for 1 more minute.
11. Assemble the burgers by placing a burger on the bottom bun, topping with bacon, tomato, and a fried egg.

Classic American Burger

Servings: 4
Cooking Time: 12 Minutes

Ingredients:

- 2 lbs ground beef
- 1/2 tsp salt
- 1/4 tsp pepper
- 4 slices American cheese
- 4 hamburger buns
- Green Leaf Lettuce
- Sliced Tomato
- Ketchup
- Mustard
- Sliced Pickle

Directions:

1. Form ground beef into four patties and season both sides with salt and pepper.
2. Grilling:
3. Preheat the grill to 500°F using direct heat with a cast iron grate installed.
4. Place burgers on the grid and close the dome for 3 minutes.
5. Flip burgers and close the dome for 2 more minutes.
6. Close all of the vents and allow the burgers to sit for 5 minutes.
7. Top each burger with a slice of cheese and close the dome for 1 more minute.
8. Build burgers with lettuce, tomato, pickle, mustard, and ketchup.

Oahu Burger

Servings: 4
Cooking Time: 12 Minutes

Ingredients:

- 2 lbs ground beef
- 1/4 cup thickened Teriyaki Marinade
- 1/4 cup mayonnaise
- 1/2 tsp sambal or sriracha
- 4 slices fresh pineapple, cored
- 4 slices tomato
- 4 slices butter lettuce
- 4 Hawaiian hamburger buns

Directions:

1. Form ground beef into four patties and season both sides with salt and pepper.
2. In a small bowl, mix mayonnaise with hot chile sauce and spread on buns.
3. Top each bun with a burger, slice of pineapple, lettuce and tomato.
4. Grilling:
5. Preheat the grill to 500°F using direct heat with a cast iron grate installed.
6. Place burgers on the grid and close the dome for 3 minutes.
7. Flip burgers, baste with Teriyaki Marinade, and place the pineapple slices on the grid. Close the dome for 2 more minutes.
8. Flip the burgers again and baste with remaining Teriyaki Marinade. Close the dome.
9. Close all of the vents and allow the burgers to sit for 5 minutes.

Quesadilla Burger

Servings: 4

Cooking Time: 12 Minutes

Ingredients:

- 2 lbs ground beef
- 2 Tablespoons Adobo Rub
- 1 cup shredded cheddar cheese
- 4 large flour tortillas
- Sour Cream
- Guacamole
- Salsa

Directions:

1. Form ground beef into four patties and season both sides with Adobo Rub.
2. Serve each burger with sour cream, guacamole, and salsa.
3. Grilling:
4. Preheat the grill to 500°F using direct heat with a cast iron grate installed.
5. Place burgers on the grid and close the dome for 3 minutes.
6. Flip burgers and close the dome for 2 more minutes.
7. Close all of the vents and allow the burgers to sit for 5 minutes.
8. Remove burgers and place flour tortillas on the grid.
9. Top each tortilla with shredded cheese and close the dome for 1 minute until the cheese melts.
10. Place a hamburger in the center of each tortilla and begin folding the tortilla around the burger like an envelope.

The Crowned Jewels Burger

Servings: 4

Cooking Time: 12 Minutes

Ingredients:

- 2 lbs ground beef
- 1/2 tsp salt
- 1/4 tsp pepper
- 1 lb thinly sliced pastrami
- 1 cup shredded Romaine lettuce
- 1/4 cup mayonnaise
- 2 Tablespoons ketchup
- 1/8 tsp onion powder
- 4 slices Sharp Cheddar cheese
- 4 hamburger buns
- 1 tomato, sliced

Directions:

1. Form ground beef into four patties and season both sides with salt and pepper.
2. Meanwhile, mix together mayonnaise, ketchup, and onion powder. Smear on each bun.
3. Place each pastrami and cheese covered burger on the prepared buns and top with shredded lettuce and tomato.
4. Grilling:
5. Preheat the grill to 500°F using direct heat with a cast iron grate installed.
6. Place burgers on the grid and close the dome for 3 minutes.
7. Flip burgers and close the dome for 2 more minutes.
8. Close all of the vents and allow the burgers to sit for 5 minutes.
9. Top each burger with 1/4 of the pastrami and a slice of cheese and close the dome for 1 more minute.

"the Masterpiece"

Servings: 4
Cooking Time: 12 Minutes

Ingredients:

- 2 lbs ground beef
- 6 ounces sliced mushrooms
- 4 Tablespoons shredded smoked Gouda
- 2 Tablespoons butter
- 2 Tablespoons olive oil
- 2 Tablespoons Dijon mustard
- 1/2 tsp salt
- 1/4 tsp pepper
- 8 slices bacon, cooked and crumbled
- 4 slices Swiss cheese
- 4 brioche buns
- 1 small onion, sliced

Directions:

1. Heat a skillet over medium heat and add 1 Tablespoon butter and 1 Tablespoon olive oil.
2. Place mushrooms in the pan and DO NOT MOVE THEM. Saute for 5-7 minutes or until the mushrooms are browned. Remove from the pan and set aside.
3. In the same skillet, heat remaining butter and olive oil and add onions. Saute over medium heat until they become translucent and begin to brown, about 10 minutes. Remove from the heat and set aside to cool.
4. Mix onion, mushrooms, and crumbled bacon.
5. Grilling:
6. Preheat the grill to 425°F using direct heat with a cast iron grate installed.
7. Form ground beef into eight patties and season both sides with salt and pepper.
8. Place a generous spoonful of the mushroom and onion mixture in the center of four patties and top with smoked Gouda.
9. Top with additional patty and press sides to seal the mixture inside.
10. Place burgers on the grid and close the dome for 5 minutes.
11. Flip burgers and close the dome for 3 more minutes.
12. Close all of the vents and allow the burgers to sit for 5 minutes.
13. Top each burger with a slice of Swiss cheese and close the dome for 1 more minute.
14. Spread buns with mustard, top with burgers and bun tops.

DESSERTS

Grilled Fruit Pie

Servings: 8
Cooking Time: 55 Minutes

Ingredients:

- for the crust
- 1 cup all-purpose flour, plus extra for rolling dough
- 1/2 tsp kosher salt
- 1/2 cup butter, chilled and cut into small cubes
- 1/4 cup ice water
- 2lb (1kg) dried beans, for blind baking
- powdered sugar, for dusting
- whipped cream or ice cream, to serve (optional)
- for the filling
- 1 1/4lb (565g) seasonal fruit, such as pears and plums, halved and pitted
- 1/2 cup sugar
- 4 tbsp cornstarch
- 2 tbsp lemon juice

Directions:

1. Preheat the grill to 350°F (177°C) using indirect heat with a standard grate installed. Place fruit on the grate skin side up, keeping them toward the edges of the grate. Close the lid and grill until beginning to soften, about 3 to 5 minutes. Transfer to a cutting board and slice. Set aside.

2. To make the crust, in a food processor, combine flour and salt, pulsing 3 to 4 times. Add butter, and pulse until the texture is mealy, about 5 to 6 times. With the food processor running, slowly add the ice water in 1 tbsp increments until the dough comes together.

3. Turn out the dough onto a floured work surface and sprinkle with flour. Using a rolling pin, roll dough out to a 10- to 11-in (25- to 28-cm) circle. Carefully transfer the dough to a 9-in (23-cm) metal pie pan, pressing the dough to the edges. Trim any overhang and crimp the edges. Prick the dough with a fork to prevent bubbles during baking. Place the pan in the fridge to chill for 15 minutes.

4. Spread a large piece of parchment paper over the dough and fill the pan with dry beans, pressing them into the edges of the dough. Place the pan on the grate, close the lid, and bake for 10 minutes. Remove the parchment and beans from the pan, and continue baking pie crust until golden brown in color, about 10 to 15 minutes more. Remove the pan from the grill and let the crust cool completely before filling.

5. To make the filling, in a large bowl, combine sugar, cornstarch, and juice. Add the grilled fruit and toss lightly to coat. Pour the fruit mixture into the baked crust. Place on the grate, close the lid, and bake until the filling is thickened and bubbling at the edges, about 30 minutes.

6. Remove the pie from the grill and place on a wire rack to cool. Just before serving, sprinkle with powdered sugar. Serve with whipped cream or ice cream (if desired).

Berry Upside-down Cake

Servings: 10
Cooking Time: 30 Minutes

Ingredients:

- 10 tbsp unsalted butter, at room temperature, divided
- 1 cup packed light brown sugar, divided
- 11oz (315g) fresh seasonal berries
- 1 large egg
- 1 tsp pure vanilla extract
- 2/3 cup sour cream
- 1 1/3 cups all-purpose flour
- 1 tbsp baking powder
- 1/4 tsp baking soda
- 1/2 tsp kosher salt
- 1/4 tsp ground cinnamon
- fresh mint leaves, to garnish
- whipped cream, to serve

Directions:

1. Preheat the grill to 350°F (177°C) using indirect heat with a standard grate installed and a cast iron skillet on the grate. Melt 2 tbsp butter in the skillet and swirl to coat. Remove the skillet from the grill. Sprinkle 1/3 cup brown sugar over butter, pour in berries, and shake the skillet until berries are evenly spread out. Set aside.

2. In the bowl of a stand mixer fitted with the paddle attachment, cream together remaining 8 tbsp butter and 2/3 cup brown sugar until fluffy. Add egg, vanilla, and sour cream, and beat to combine.

3. In a medium bowl, sift together flour, baking powder, baking soda, salt, and cinnamon. Gradually add the dry ingredients to the butter and egg mixture until just incorporated. (The batter will be thick.) Using a rubber spatula, scoop the batter into the skillet, smoothing it over berries.

4. Place the skillet on the grate, close the lid, and bake until golden brown and a cake tester inserted into the middle of the cake comes out clean, about 30 minutes. Remove the skillet from the grill and place on a wire rack to cool for 15 minutes.

5. To serve, flip the cake upside down on a large serving platter and release from the skillet, leaving the berries on top. Garnish with fresh mint leaves, and serve with a dollop of whipped cream.

Corn & Jalapeño Focaccia

Servings: 8

Cooking Time: 40 Minutes

Ingredients:

- 2 1/2 cups all-purpose or bread flour
- 1 tbsp kosher salt
- 1/2 tbsp instant dry yeast
- 1 1/2 cups warm water (105°F [41°C])
- 3 tbsp extra virgin olive oil
- 3 jalapeño peppers, left whole
- 1 ear of corn, shucked

- for the butter
- 1 tbsp olive oil
- 2 tbsp unsalted butter
- 4 garlic cloves, minced
- 2 tsp dried oregano
- 1/2 tsp red pepper flakes
- kosher salt

Directions:

1. In a large bowl, combine flour, salt, yeast, and water. Cover tightly with plastic wrap, and set aside to rest for at least 8 hours and up to 24 hours. The dough will rise dramatically and fill the bowl.

2. Pour oil into a large cast iron skillet. Transfer the dough to the skillet, turning the dough to coat in oil. Press the dough around the skillet, flattening slightly and spreading to fill the entire bottom. Cover tightly with plastic wrap and let sit at room temperature for 2 hours.

3. After the first hour, preheat the grill to 425°F (218°C) using indirect heat with a standard grate installed. Place jalapeños and corn on the grate near the edges. Close the lid and grill until beginning to soften and char, about 10 to 12 minutes. Cut the kernels from the cob, and seed and dice jalapeños. Set aside.

4. After resting for 2 hours, the dough should mostly fill the skillet. Use your fingertips to firmly press the dough to the edges, popping any large bubbles that appear. Lift the dough at the edges and allow any air bubbles underneath to escape.

5. Evenly scatter corn and jalapeños over the dough, then push down until they're embedded in the dough. Place the skillet on the grate, close the grill lid, and bake until the top is golden brown and the bottom appears golden brown and crisp when lifted at the edge with a spatula, about 16 to 24 minutes.

6. To make the butter, on the stovetop in a small saucepan over medium-low heat, heat oil and butter until butter melts. Add garlic, oregano, and pepper flakes, and cook for 1 minute, stirring constantly. Transfer to a small bowl and season with salt to taste.

7. Transfer the focaccia to a cutting board and brush the butter over top. Allow to cool slightly, slice, and serve with any remaining butter.

Seasonal Fruit Cobbler

Servings: 12
Cooking Time: 90 Minutes

Ingredients:

- 2lb (1kg) seasonal fruit, washed, pitted (if needed), and sliced or halved if needed
- 1/2 tsp ground cinnamon
- 2 tsp cornstarch (for juicy fruits; omit for pears or apples)
- 4 tbsp butter, plus more for greasing
- 1/2 cup sugar, plus more for sprinkling
- 3/4 cup self-rising flour
- 3/4 cup whole milk
- whipped cream, to serve

Directions:

1. Preheat the grill to 350°F (177°C) using indirect heat with a standard grate installed. Place the fruit on the grate (or in a cast iron skillet if the fruit might fall through the grate), close the lid, and grill until beginning to soften and char, about 7 to 10 minutes. Remove fruit from the grill and place in a large bowl. Sprinkle cinnamon and cornstarch (if using) over fruit, and add a little sugar (if desired). Gently toss to coat and set aside.
2. Grease a 9-in (23-cm) grill-safe baking pan with butter. On the stovetop in a small saucepan, heat 4 tbsp butter over medium-low heat until beginning to brown, about 10 to 15 minutes.
3. In a medium bowl, whisk together butter, sugar, flour, and milk. Transfer fruit to the prepared baking pan and spread the batter evenly over top. Place the pan on the grate, close the lid, and bake until golden brown and bubbly, about 1 hour. In the last 10 minutes of cooking, sprinkle a light amount of sugar over top. Remove the cobbler from the grill, and serve warm with whipped cream on top.

Chocolate Chip Cookie Peanut Butter Cup S'mores

Servings: 4
Cooking Time: 5 Minutes

Ingredients:

- 8 chocolate chip cookies
- 4 peanut butter cup candies
- 4 marshmallows

Directions:

1. On the grid of a 225°F grill, place one cookie, flat side up, with one peanut butter cup candy and one marshmallow on top.
2. Close the dome for 5 minutes or until the marshmallow begins to puff.
3. Assembly:
4. Close the s'more with the other chocolate chip cookie and get ready for the sugar rush.

Fresh Peach Crisp

Servings: 4

Cooking Time: 5 Minutes

Ingredients:

- 2 peaches, halved with pits removed
- Vanilla Ice Cream
- 1 cup good quality granola

Directions:

1. Grilling:
2. Place the peach halves, cut side down, on a 400°F grill and cover with the dome for 5 minutes.
3. Assembly:
4. Remove the peaches and place them, cut side up, in a bowl. Top with vanilla ice cream and granola.

Brownies

Servings: 6

Cooking Time: 30 Minutes

Ingredients:

- 1 1/2 cups flour
- 1 cup white sugar
- 1 cup brown sugar
- 3/4 cups cocoa powder
- 1/2 cup butter, melted
- 1/4 cup vegetable oil
- 2 tsp vanilla
- 1 tsp baking powder
- 1/2 tsp salt
- 4 eggs
- 1/2 cup chocolate chips
- 1/2 chip marshmallows

Directions:

1. In a large bowl, combine butter, oil and sugars.
2. Add eggs, one at a time, stirring in between.
3. Add vanilla and stir.
4. Sift together cocoa powder, baking powder, and flour.
5. Add to the butter and egg mixture and stir until just combined.
6. Grilling:
7. Preheat the grill to 350°F using direct heat with a cast iron grate installed.
8. Line the dutch oven with a liner.
9. Pour the batter into the liner.
10. Cover the dutch oven, place on the grid, and lower the dome for 25-30 minutes or until a toothpick inserted into the middle comes out clean.
11. Remove the lid, top the brownies with chocolate chips and marshmallows and replace the lid for 5 minutes until the toppings are melted.

Pizza Margherita

Servings: 2

Cooking Time: 6 Minutes

Ingredients:

- cornmeal, for dusting
- 1/4 cup marinara sauce
- 2oz (55g) fresh mozzarella, sliced
- 3 garlic cloves, thinly sliced
- 12–16 fresh basil leaves
- kosher salt and freshly ground black pepper
- grated Parmesan, to serve
- for the dough
- 12oz (340g) Italian 00 flour, plus more for dusting
- 4 tsp kosher salt
- 2 tsp instant dry yeast
- 61/2oz (190ml) warm water (105°F [41°C])

Directions:

1. To make the dough, in a large bowl, whisk together flour, salt, and yeast until well combined. Add water, and use your hands to mix until no dry flour remains. Cover tightly with plastic wrap and allow to rise at room temperature for 2 to 4 hours. Turn the dough out onto a lightly floured surface and allow to sit at room temperature for 2 hours before baking.

2. Preheat the grill to 600°F (316°C) using indirect heat with a pizza stone resting directly on the heat deflector. (The pizza stone should be level with the grill rim.)

3. On a lightly floured work surface, roll out the dough to 1/4 in (.5cm) thick and a 10-in (25cm) diameter. Lightly dust a pizza paddle or unrimmed baking sheet with cornmeal, and place the dough on top. Evenly spread the sauce over the dough, working from the center to the edges. Top with the sliced mozzarella and garlic.

4. Carefully slide the pizza from the paddle to the hot pizza stone. Close the lid and bake until the crust is golden brown and the cheese is melted and beginning to bubble, about 4 to 6 minutes.

5. Use the pizza paddle to remove the pizza from the grill. Scatter the basil leaves over top and sprinkle with salt, pepper, and Parmesan.

Caramel Cinnamon Rolls

Servings: 4
Cooking Time: 30 Minutes

Ingredients:

- 18 frozen cinnamon rolls, thawed (you can also used canned cinnamon rolls)
- 1/2 cup brown sugar
- 1/2 cup graham cracker crumbs
- 1/2 cup caramel ice cream topping
- 1 tsp cinnamon

Directions:

1. Line the dutch oven with a liner.
2. Cut each cinnamon roll into 4 pieces and arrange them around the bottom of the dutch oven.
3. In a separate bowl, combine brown sugar, graham cracker crumbs, and cinnamon.
4. Sprinkle some of the mixture over the layer of cinnamon rolls. Repeat.
5. Grilling:
6. Preheat the grill to 350°F using direct heat with a cast iron grate installed.
7. Cover the dutch oven and place it on the grid of the grill.
8. Lower the dome for 25-30 minutes or until the cinnamon rolls are golden brown.
9. Drizzle caramel ice cream topping over the warm rolls and serve.

Grilled Sopapillas

Servings: 6
Cooking Time: 18 Minutes

Ingredients:

- 1 pizza dough, divided into 6 pieces
- 3 Tablespoons melted butter
- 1/4 cup sugar
- 1 Tablespoon cinnamon

Directions:

1. Stretch dough into round shape.
2. Place the dough directly on the pizza stone in a 500°F grill.
3. Brush with melted butter and top with cinnamon sugar.
4. Close the dome for 3 minutes, then remove.
5. Repeat with remaining dough.

Whole Apples With Caramel Sauce

Servings: 4

Cooking Time: 60 Minutes

Ingredients:

- 4 Jonathan Apples
- 1 cup packed dark brown sugar
- 1/2 cup half and half
- 4 Tablespoons butter
- 1 tsp vanilla extract

Directions:

1. In a medium saucepan, whisk together the brown sugar, butter, and half and half until melted.
2. Continue whisking 5-7 minutes until the caramel begins to thicken.
3. Add vanilla and set aside to cool before storing in a jar in the fridge.
4. Using a melon baller, scoop the core from the apple.
5. Wrap each apple in aluminum foil.
6. Grilling:
7. Preheat the grill to 225°F using direct heat with a cast iron grate installed for 1 hour.
8. Remove apples from the grill, serve topped with caramel sauce.

Almond Cream Cake

Servings: 16
Cooking Time: 45 Minutes

Ingredients:

- 2 cups butter, softened
- 3 cups sugar
- 6 cups cake flour
- 1 tsp kosher salt
- 4 tsp baking powder
- 2 cups whole milk
- 2 tsp almond extract
- 10 large eggs, whites only
- sliced almonds, to decorate
- for the frosting
- 1 1/4 cups all-purpose flour
- 2 cups whole milk
- 1/2 tsp almond extract
- 1 tbsp vanilla bean paste
- 2 cups butter, softened
- 2 cups sugar

Directions:

1. In the bowl of a stand mixer fitted with the paddle attachment, cream butter until white in appearance. Add sugar and beat until fluffy. In a large bowl, sift together flour, salt, and baking powder. Add the flour mixture to the butter mixture in three stages, alternating with the milk and almond extract and mixing after each addition until just combined.

2. In a large bowl, beat egg whites until they form stiff peaks. Using a spatula, gently fold egg whites into the cake batter, taking care not to overmix.

3. Preheat the grill to 350°F (177°C) using indirect heat with a standard grate installed. Line an 11 x18-in (28 x 46cm) grill-safe baking pan with parchment paper and lightly grease with cooking spray. Pour the batter into the pan, place on the grate, close the lid, and bake until the top springs back when touched, about 27 to 30 minutes.

4. Remove the cake from the grill and place on a wire rack to cool for 10 minutes. Use a knife to loosen the edges, and transfer the cake to a wire rack to cool completely.

5. To make the frosting, on the stovetop in a saucepan over medium-low heat, whisk together flour and milk until mixture thickens to the consistency of mashed potatoes, about 12 to 15 minutes. Stir constantly, and lower the heat if needed. Remove the saucepan from the heat and place in a bowl of ice for 5 to 10 minutes to hasten the cooling process and bring the mixture to room temperature. Once cool, stir in almond extract.

6. In the bowl of a stand mixer, cream together vanilla paste, butter, and sugar until the mixture is light and fluffy and sugar is completely dissolved. Add the flour mixture, and beat until it has the appearance of whipped cream, scraping the sides of the bowl as needed.

7. Spread the frosting evenly over the cooled cake and sprinkle sliced almonds over top to decorate before serving.

Peaches And Pound Cake

Servings: 6
Cooking Time: 5 Minutes

Ingredients:

- 1/2 cup heavy whipping cream
- 2 Tablespoons sour cream
- 3 peaches, halved and pitted
- 1 store-bought pound cake, cut into 6 slices

Directions:

1. Place the peaches, cut side down, on a 400°F grill.
2. Place the pound cake slices alongside the peaches and close the dome for 2 minutes.
3. Flip the pound cake, and close the dome for an additional 2-3 minutes.
4. Assembly:
5. In a stand mixer, whip the whipping cream until stiff peaks form. Fold in the sour cream to combine.
6. Place a slice of pound cake on a plate, top with a peach half, and a dollop of the cream.

3 Ingredient Fruit Cobbler

Servings: 8
Cooking Time: 30 Minutes

Ingredients:

- 1 stick butter, sliced
- 2 (29 oz) cans fruit, drained but reserving 1/2 cup of the liquid
- 1 yellow cake mix

Directions:

1. Line the dutch oven with a liner
2. Pour fruit into the bottom of the dutch oven with 1/2 cup of reserved liquid
3. Sprinkle the top with cake mix
4. Dot the top with butter.
5. Grilling:
6. Preheat the grill to 350°F using direct heat with a cast iron grate installed.
7. Cover the dutch oven and place on the grid of the grill.
8. Lower the dome for 30 minutes.
9. Allow the cobbler to sit for 10 minutes off the heat before serving.

Grilled Plums With Honey And Ricotta

Servings: 4

Cooking Time: 5 Minutes

Ingredients:

- 4 plums, cut in half and pitted
- 1/2 cup whole milk ricotta cheese
- 2 Tablespoons honey
- 1/4 tsp cracked black pepper

Directions:

1. Place the plums, cut side down on a 400°F grill.
2. Close the dome for 5 minutes.
3. Assembly:
4. Serve the plums, cut side up, with a dollop of ricotta, a drizzle of honey, and a sprinkling of cracked black pepper.

Grilled Naan

Servings: 24

Cooking Time: 6 Minutes

Ingredients:

- 1 cup warm water (105°F [41°C])
- 1/4oz (7g) active dry yeast
- 1/4 cup sugar
- 3 tbsp whole milk
- 1 large egg, beaten
- 2 tsp kosher salt
- 20¼oz (575g) bread flour, plus more for kneading
- vegetable oil, for greasing
- 1/4 cup butter, melted

Directions:

1. In a large bowl, combine water and yeast. Let sit until frothy, about 10 minutes. Stir in sugar, milk, egg, salt, and flour to make a soft dough. Knead on a lightly floured surface until smooth.
2. Lightly oil a large bowl, place the dough in the bowl, and cover with a damp cloth. Let sit to rise until the dough has doubled in volume, about 1 hour.
3. Punch the dough down and divide it into 4 balls (about the size of golf balls). Cover with a towel and allow to rise until the balls have doubled in size, about 30 minutes.
4. Preheat the grill to 425°F (218°C) using direct heat with a cast iron grate installed. Use a rolling pin one ball of dough into a thin circle. Lightly oil the grate, place the circle of dough on the grate, close the lid, and bake until puffy and lightly browned, about 2 to 3 minutes. Brush the uncooked side with butter, then flip the dough over and brush the cooked side with butter. Cook until puffy and lightly browned, about 3 minutes more. Repeat the cooking process with the remaining dough. (You can also bake all 4 balls at the same time.)
5. Remove the naan from the grill and sprinkle with seasoning of choice (if desired). Serve warm.

Upside Down Triple Berry Pie

Servings: 8
Cooking Time: 35 Minutes

Ingredients:

- 6 cups frozen triple berry mix
- 2 Tablespoons lemon juice
- 1 refrigerated pie crust
- 1 cup sugar, divided
- 4 Tablespoons cornstarch

Directions:

1. Place a liner in the dutch oven.
2. In a separate bowl, combine frozen berries with 3/4 cup sugar, cornstarch, and lemon juice.
3. Pour berries into the bottom of the lined dutch oven.
4. Unroll pie crust and place on top of berry mixture.
5. Cut 4 vent holes into the crust.
6. Sprinkle remaining sugar over the pie crust.
7. Grilling:
8. Preheat the grill to 425°F using direct heat with a cast iron grate installed.
9. Cover the dutch oven and place on the grid.
10. Lower the dome for 35 minutes or until the crust is golden and the berry mixture has thickened.
11. Cut the crust as you would any pie.
12. Serve a piece of crust topped with ice cream and a scoop of the thickened berry mixture.

Death By Chocolate

Servings: 8
Cooking Time: 60 Minutes

Ingredients:

- 1 chocolate cake mix, prepared according to package directions
- 2 cups chocolate chips
- 1 cup brown sugar
- 1 1/2 cups water
- 1/2 cup cocoa powder
- 1 (10 oz) bag miniature marshmallows

Directions:

1. Prepare cake mix according to package instructions.
2. Line the dutch oven with a liner.
3. In a medium bowl, combine water, brown sugar, and cocoa powder.
4. Pour the mixture into the bottom of the dutch oven.
5. Top with miniature marshmallows
6. Pour prepared cake mix on top.
7. Top with chocolate chips.
8. Grilling:
9. Preheat the grill to 350°F using direct heat with a cast iron grate installed.
10. Place the lid on the dutch oven and set on the grid of the grill.
11. Close the dome for 1 hour.
12. Remove the dutch oven from the grill, uncover, and serve warm.

Sourdough Baguette

Servings: 4

Cooking Time: 25 Minutes

Ingredients:

- cornmeal, for dusting
- for Day 1 (starter)
- 8oz (225g) whole rye flour
- 8oz (235ml) warm water (105°F [41°C])
- for Day 2
- 8oz (225g) bread flour
- for Day 3
- 12oz (340g) bread flour
- 6oz (177ml) warm water (105°F [41°C])

- 8oz (225g) starter
- for Day 4
- 3oz (85g) whole rye flour
- 31oz (915ml) warm water (105°F [41°C])
- 9½oz (270g) starter
- 42oz (1.2kg) bread flour
- 3oz (85g) whole wheat flour
- 1oz (25g) kosher salt

Directions:

1. On Day 1, in a large bowl, combine flour and water, cover tightly with plastic wrap, and let sit overnight on the counter at warm room temperature, about 70°F (21°C). (Cooler temperatures might inhibit the growth of the starter.)

2. On Day 2, add flour to the starter and mix until a stiff, thick dough forms. Cover tightly with plastic wrap and let sit overnight on the counter at warm room temperature. The dough will rise overnight.

3. On Day 3, in a large bowl, combine flour, water, and 8 ounces (225g) of the starter, and mix until a stiff, thick dough forms. Cover tightly with plastic wrap and let sit overnight on the counter at warm room temperature. The dough will rise overnight and should begin to smell yeasty. (Freeze remaining starter for later use.)

4. On Day 4, preheat the grill to 400°F (204°C) using indirect heat with a standard grate installed and a pizza stone on the grate. In a large bowl, combine rye flour, water, 9½ ounces (270g) of the starter, bread flour, wheat flour, and salt, and mix until a dough forms. Cover tightly with plastic wrap and let sit for 20 minutes on the counter. The dough will continue to smell yeasty. (Freeze remaining starter for later use.)

5. Form the dough into 4 baguette shapes that are 10 to 12 inches (25cm to 30.5cm) long and about 2½ inches (6.25cm) around. Make 3 slits in the top of each loaf to allow steam to escape. Sprinkle the pizza stone with cornmeal and place the loaves on the pizza stone. Close the lid and bake until the bread reaches an internal temperature of 190°F (88°C), about 20 to 25 minutes.

6. Remove the baguettes from the grill, place on a cutting board, and let rest before slicing and serving as desired.

Lemon Poppy Seed Cake

Servings: 10

Cooking Time: 45 Minutes

Ingredients:

- 1 tsp poppy seeds
- 2 lemons, zested and juiced
- 1 vanilla cake mix prepared according to package directions, substituting melted butter for oil and buttermilk for water
- 1 lb powdered sugar
- 4 ounces cream cheese
- 1 stick butter, softened
- 1/2 tsp vanilla
- 1/2 tsp lemon extract
- The juice and zest of 1 lemon

Directions:

1. Prepare cake mix according to package directions, substituting melted butter for the oil and buttermilk for the water.
2. Add the lemon zest, lemon juice, and poppy seeds.
3. Line the dutch oven with a liner.
4. Pour prepare cake mix into the liner and cover.
5. Grilling:
6. Preheat the grill to 350°F using direct heat with a cast iron grate installed.
7. Place the dutch oven on the grid and lower the dome for 30-40 minutes or until a toothpick inserted into the center comes out clean.
8. Meanwhile, combine glaze ingredients, adding milk to thin out the glaze if necessary.
9. Remove the cake from the grill and set aside to cool for 10 minutes before pouring glaze over the cake.
10. Serve warm.

Best Banana Bread

Servings: 6

Cooking Time: 40 Minutes

Ingredients:

- 1 cup plain yogurt
- 1/4 cup butter
- 3 very ripe bananas, peeled
- 2 eggs
- 2 cups flour

- 2/3 cups sugar
- 3/4 tsp salt
- 1/2 tsp vanilla extract
- 1/2 tsp baking soda
- 1/4 tsp baking powder

Directions:

1. In a blender, combine bananas, yogurt, sugar, butter, vanilla, and eggs until smooth.
2. In a large bowl, sift together flour, salt, baking powder, and baking soda.
3. Gradually add the wet ingredients into the dry ingredients and gently stir to combine. DO NOT OVER MIX.
4. Line a dutch oven with a liner.
5. Pour batter into the dutch oven and cover.
6. Grilling:
7. Preheat the grill to 350°F using direct heat with a cast iron grate installed and place the dutch oven on the grid.
8. Lower the dome for 30 minutes or until a toothpick inserted into the center comes out clean.

Peach Dutch Baby

Servings: 8

Cooking Time: 25 Minutes

Ingredients:

- 8 oz frozen peaches, thawed (or 3 ripe peaches, peeled and sliced)
- 1 cup whole milk
- 4 eggs
- 1 cup flour

- 1/4 cup sugar
- 1/4 cup butter
- 1 tsp vanilla
- 1 tsp cinnamon
- 1/2 tsp salt

Directions:

1. In a blender, combine milk, flour, sugar, vanilla, cinnamon, salt, and eggs until smooth.
2. Grilling:
3. Preheat the grill to 425°F using direct heat with a cast iron grate installed.
4. Place the dutch oven on the grid of the grill and melt the butter.
5. Line the bottom of the pot with peaches and pour over milk and egg mixture.
6. Close the dome for 20 minutes or until the top of the Dutch Baby is golden brown.
7. Serve with a sprinkling of powdered sugar.

Apple Cake

Servings: 12
Cooking Time: 60 Minutes

Ingredients:

- 2 (21 oz) cans apple pie filling
- 1 (14 oz) jar caramel ice cream topping
- 1 box yellow cake mix, prepared according to package directions and mixed with 2 tsp cinnamon

Directions:

1. Prepare cake according to package directions.
2. Line a dutch oven with a liner.
3. Pour pie filling into the bottom of the dutch oven.
4. Top with caramel ice cream topping.
5. Top with prepared cake mix.
6. Grilling:
7. Preheat the grill to 350°F using direct heat with a cast iron grate installed.
8. Cover the dutch oven and place on the grid of the grill.
9. Lower the dome and cook for 1 hour.
10. Serve warm with whipped cream or ice cream.

Peanut Butter Bacon Bars

Servings: 8
Cooking Time: 25 Minutes

Ingredients:

- 1 package peanut butter cookie mix
- 1/2 cup chopped peanuts
- 1/2 cup bacon, cooked and crumbled
- 1/3 cup vegetable oil
- 1 egg
- 1 cup semi-sweet chocolate chips
- 1/2 cup bacon, cooked and crumbled

Directions:

1. Combine cookie mix, vegetable oil, egg, bacon, and peanuts and press into a lined dutch oven.
2. Grilling:
3. Preheat the grill to 350°F using direct heat with a cast iron grate installed.
4. Cover the dutch oven and place on the grid.
5. Lower the dome for 25 minutes.
6. Remove the lid and top with chocolate chips.
7. Replace the cover for 5 minutes until the chocolate chips are melted.
8. Spread the chocolate over the bars to coat them evenly.
9. Top with remaining bacon.
10. Allow the bars to cool before cutting.

SIDES

Soba Noodle Bowl

Servings: 6
Cooking Time: 30 Minutes

Ingredients:

- 12oz (28g) soba noodles
- 4 scallions
- 2 red bell peppers, left whole
- 1 carrot, peeled
- 1/2 head of napa cabbage
- 1/4 cup chopped hazelnuts
- chopped fresh cilantro, to garnish
- for the sauce
- 1/2 cup peanut butter
- 1/4 cup soy sauce
- 1/3 cup warm water
- 2 tbsp ground ginger
- 1 garlic clove
- 2 tbsp white wine vinegar
- 11/2 tsp honey
- 1 tsp crushed red pepper flakes

Directions:

1. To make the sauce, combine all the sauce ingredients in a blender and purée until smooth. Set aside. (Sauce can be made in advance. Refrigerate in an airtight container and use within 1 week.)

2. Cook the pasta according to the package directions until cooked but still firm to the bite. Drain and rinse well under cold water. Set aside.

3. Preheat the grill to 400°F (204°C) using direct heat with a cast iron grate installed and a cast iron skillet on the grate. Place scallions, peppers, carrot, and napa cabbage around the skillet, close the lid, and grill until beginning to soften and char, about 7 to 10 minutes. Slice peppers and carrots thinly, and shred cabbage.

4. Add the vegetables and noodles to the hot skillet, and stir to combine. Add the sauce, and stir until well incorporated and heated through, about 3 to 4 minutes.

5. Remove the skillet from the grill and top noodles with hazelnuts and cilantro. Serve immediately.

Prosciutto And Pear Bruschetta

Servings: 6
Cooking Time: 5 Minutes

Ingredients:
- 4 oz prosciutto
- 4 oz shaved parmesan cheese
- 1 cup baby arugula
- 1 baguette, sliced 1/2 inch thick
- 1 pear, sliced thin
- 2 Tablespoons olive oil
- 2 Tablespoons high quality balsamic vinegar

Directions:
1. Brush each baguette slice with olive oil and place on a 325°F grill with the dome closed for 5 minutes.
2. Assembly:
3. Remove bread slices and top each with prosciutto, pear slices, parmesan, and baby arugula.
4. Drizzle a few drops of balsamic vinegar over each bruschetta and serve.

Broiled Tomatoes And Parmesan

Servings: 4
Cooking Time: 5 Minutes

Ingredients:
- 1/4 cup parmesan, shredded
- 4 roma tomatoes
- 1 Tablespoon olive oil
- 1 tsp red wine vinegar
- Salt & Pepper

Directions:
1. Cut each tomato in half, lengthwise, and brush with olive oil.
2. Grilling:
3. Preheat the grill to 500°F using direct heat with a cast iron grate installed and lower the dome for 2 minutes.
4. Turn the tomatoes, season with vinegar, salt, and pepper and top with parmesan cheese.
5. Lower the dome for an additional 2 minutes or until the cheese melts. Serve warm.

Lasagna

Servings: 12

Cooking Time: 75 Minutes

Ingredients:

- 2 cups ricotta cheese
- 1 cup mozzarella cheese
- 1/2 cup grated parmesan cheese
- 1 egg
- 1 tsp Italian seasoning
- 2 jars (24 oz) marinara sauce or 1 recipe Bolognese sauce
- 1 package no-boil lasagna noodles

Directions:

1. In a medium sized bowl, combine ricotta, parmesan, Italian seasoning, and egg.

2. In a lined dutch oven, pour 1 cup marinara sauce into the bottom of the pot. Layer noodles, ricotta mixture, and sauce in repeating layers ending with sauce.

3. Grilling:

4. Preheat the grill to 350°F using direct heat with a cast iron grate installed.

5. Cover the dutch oven and place it in the grill for 1 hour.

6. Remove from the grill, uncover, and top with mozzarella cheese.

7. Recover the dutch oven and allow the lasagna to sit for 5 more minutes before uncovering.

8. Allow the lasagna to rest for 10 minutes before serving.

9. Traditional Spanish Paella has rabbit, small clams, and chorizo in it. Cubans use lobster, shrimp, and chicken. This version is a combination of the two but the protein is really a matter of taste.

Roasted Potatoes

Servings: 20

Cooking Time: 30 Minutes

Ingredients:

- 2lb (1kg) fingerling potatoes, halved
- 1 tbsp chopped fresh cilantro
- 1 tbsp chopped fresh basil
- 1 tbsp chopped scallions, plus more to garnish
- 3 poblano peppers, diced
- 1/2 cup olive oil
- 1/2 cup white vinegar
- 3 garlic cloves, minced
- kosher salt and freshly ground black pepper
- 1 cup crumbled queso fresco

Directions:

1. Preheat the grill to 425°F (218°C) using indirect heat with a standard grate installed. In a dutch oven or a disposable aluminum baking dish, combine potatoes, cilantro, basil, scallions, peppers, oil, vinegar, and garlic. Toss well to ensure potatoes are coated in oil and seasonings. Place the dutch oven on the grate and cook until potatoes are fork tender, about 30 minutes.

2. Remove the dutch oven from the grill, season with salt and pepper to taste, and top with the queso fresco and more sliced scallions. Serve immediately.

Mac And Cheese

Servings: 6

Cooking Time: 60 Minutes

Ingredients:
- 1 lb smoked cheddar cheese, shredded, divided
- 1/4 cup butter
- 2 eggs
- 1/2 lb elbow macaroni
- 3/4 cups evaporated milk
- 1/4 cup Panko breadcrumbs
- 1 tsp salt
- 3/4 tsp dry mustard

Directions:
1. In a large pot of boiling, salted water cook the macaroni according to package directions and drain.
2. In a separate bowl, whisk together the eggs, milk, hot sauce, salt, pepper, and mustard.
3. Grilling:
4. Preheat the grill to 350°F using direct heat with a cast iron grate installed with the dutch oven on the grid.
5. Melt the butter in the dutch oven and place macaroni in the pot. Toss to coat.
6. Stir the egg and milk mixture into the pasta and add half of the cheese.
7. Continuously stir the mac and cheese for 3 minutes or until creamy.
8. Top with remaining cheese and Panko breadcrumbs.
9. Cover the dutch oven, lower the dome, and cook for 20-25 minutes.
10. Serve immediately.

Summer Squash & Eggplant

Servings: 6

Cooking Time: 35 Minutes

Ingredients:

- 1 medium yellow squash
- 2 medium zucchini
- 1/4 cup olive oil
- 2 medium yellow onions, sliced into half moons
- 1 medium eggplant, peeled and cut into cubes
- 2 garlic cloves, minced
- 1/2 tsp dried oregano
- 2 cups dry white wine, such as Chardonnay
- 4 tbsp unsalted butter
- kosher salt and freshly ground black pepper
- lemon slices, to serve (optional)

Directions:

1. Preheat the grill to 425°F (218°C) using direct heat with a cast iron grate installed and a dutch oven on the grate. Place squash and zucchini on the grate around the dutch oven, close the lid, and grill until beginning to soften and char, about 5 to 7 minutes. Remove vegetables from the grill and slice into rounds.
2. In the hot dutch oven, heat oil until shimmering. Add onions, and sauté until translucent, about 7 to 8 minutes. Add squash, zucchini, eggplant, garlic, and oregano. Close the lid and sauté until vegetables begin to soften, about 15 minutes. Add white wine, close the grill lid, and simmer until the vegetables have begun to soften and the liquid has reduced by half, about 5 minutes.
3. Remove the dutch oven from the grill and add the butter, stirring until melted. Season well with salt and pepper and a squeeze of lemon. Serve hot with lemon slices (if using).

Parmesan Zucchini Spears

Servings: 4

Cooking Time: 10 Minutes

Ingredients:

- 4 zucchini, cut in half, then cut into quarters lengthwise
- 1/2 cup parmesan, grated
- 1 tsp Italian seasoning
- 1/2 tsp garlic powder
- Salt and Pepper to taste
- Olive oil for brushing

Directions:

1. Brush each zucchini spear with olive oil and season with salt and pepper.
2. In a small bowl, combine Italian seasoning, garlic powder, and parmesan.
3. Place zucchini spears on a small sheet tray and sprinkle the parmesan over each spear.
4. Grilling:
5. Place the sheet tray on the grid of a 500°F grill.
6. Close the dome and cook for 10 minutes or until the parmesan is golden brown. Serve warm.

Smoked Potato Salad

Servings: 8
Cooking Time: 120 Minutes

Ingredients:

- 4 large baking potatoes
- 4 large eggs, hard boiled and finely chopped
- 2 green onions, finely chopped
- 2 large dill pickles, finely chopped
- 1 rib celery, finely diced
- 1/2 cup mayonnaise
- The juice of 1 lemon
- 1/2 tsp black pepper
- 1/2 tsp celery seed
- 1/2 tsp dried dill

Directions:

1. Scrub the potatoes.
2. Grilling:
3. Place the potatoes alongside meat that is smoking at 225°F.
4. Assembly:
5. When the potatoes are fork tender, chill in the refrigerator for 30 minutes.
6. Peel and cut potatoes into small cubes.
7. In a large bowl, combine dressing ingredients.
8. Add potatoes, eggs, green onion, pickle, and celery to the dressing and gently toss

Sweet Potato Fries

Servings: 4
Cooking Time: 25 Minutes

Ingredients:

- 1 tsp fresh thyme, chopped
- 4 large sweet potatoes
- 4 cloves garlic, minced
- 1/4 cup olive oil
- Salt and Pepper

Directions:

1. In a large pot, cover sweet potatoes with cold water and add 2 tsp salt.
2. Bring the water to a boil and cook until the potatoes are soft, but firm, about 15 minutes.
3. In a small sauce pan, heat 2 Tablespoon of the olive oil, garlic, and thyme until fragrant.
4. Cut each sweet potato in half, lengthwise, then in 3 or 4 spears.
5. Brush each spear on cut sides with olive oil, season with salt and pepper.
6. Grilling:
7. Preheat the grill to 425°F using direct heat with a cast iron grate installed and close the dome for 3 minutes.
8. Turn the potatoes and close the dome for an additional 3 minutes or until the sweet potatoes have finished cooking through.
9. Remove the fries and toss with the garlic and thyme oil before serving.

Sweet Potato Bake

Servings: 6

Cooking Time: 20 Minutes

Ingredients:

- 3 cups cooked and mashed sweet potatoes, cooled
- 1/2 cup butter, melted
- 1/2 cup sugar
- 1/2 cup milk
- 1 tsp vanilla extract
- 1/2 tsp salt
- 3 eggs, beaten
- 1 cup brown sugar
- 1/2 cup self-rising flour
- 1 cup chopped pecans
- 4 Tablespoons butter at room temperature

Directions:

1. Line the dutch oven with a liner.
2. In a large bowl, combine souffle ingredients. Pour into the prepared dutch oven.
3. In a separate small bowl, combine brown sugar, self-rising flour, chopped pecans, and room temperature butter until a crumbly mixture forms.
4. Sprinkle the crumb mixture over the sweet potato mixture.
5. Grilling:
6. Preheat the grill to 400°F using direct heat with a cast iron grate installed.
7. Place the dutch oven, uncovered, into the grill for 20-25 minutes or until the top is golden brown.

Breakfast Casserole

Servings: 6

Cooking Time: 40 Minutes

Ingredients:

- 1 lb bulk pork breakfast sausage
- 1 (16 oz) bag of frozen O'Brien style hash browns
- 1 dozen eggs, beaten
- 1/4 cup grated onion
- 1/4 tsp black pepper
- Hot sauce for garnish

Directions:

1. Preheat the grill to 350°F using direct heat with a cast iron grate installed with the dutch oven on the grid.
2. Brown sausage with onion in the dutch oven.
3. Add hash browns and stir to combine.
4. Add eggs and cover.
5. Lower the dome for 15 minutes or until the eggs are just cooked through.
6. Serve the casserole with hot sauce for garnish.

Corn & Poblano Pudding

Servings: 8
Cooking Time: 30 Minutes

Ingredients:

- vegetable oil, for greasing
- 4 ears of sweet corn, shucked
- 1 poblano pepper, left whole
- 4 large eggs
- 1 cup whole milk
- 1/2 tsp kosher salt
- 1/4 tsp ground nutmeg
- 1/4 tsp ground cayenne pepper
- 2oz (55g) shredded Cheddar cheese

Directions:

1. Preheat the grill to 350°F (177°C) using indirect heat with a standard grate installed. Grease a cast iron skillet with oil.

2. Place corn and pepper on the grate, positioning them around the edges, close the lid, and grill until beginning to soften and char, about 10 minutes. Transfer the vegetables to a cutting board, cut the kernels from the cobs, and seed and dice the pepper.

3. In a large bowl, whisk together eggs, milk, salt, nutmeg, cayenne, and cheese until well combined. Stir in corn kernels and pepper. Pour the mixture into the greased dish and place on the grate. Close the lid and bake until a knife inserted halfway between the center and the outer edge comes out clean, about 20 minutes. Remove the pudding from the grill and serve warm or at room temperature.

Cowboy Caviar

Servings: 8
Cooking Time: 10 Minutes

Ingredients:

- 2 ears fresh corn on the cob
- 1 large tomato, finely diced
- 1 bell pepper, finely diced
- 1 jalapeño, very finely chopped
- 1/4 cup bottled Italian salad dressing
- 2 cans black beans, drained and rinsed
- 1 can pinto beans, drained and rinsed

Directions:

1. Place shucked and cleaned ears of corn on a 425°F grill and close the dome for 5 minutes.
2. Turn the corn and close the dome for another 5 minutes before removing and setting aside.
3. Assembly:
4. Carefully cut the corn off the cob and place it in a large bow.
5. Add remaining ingredients and toss to combine.

Baba Ganoush

Servings: 8

Cooking Time: 10 Minutes

Ingredients:

- 2 Tablespoons fresh parsley
- 1 eggplant, sliced into 1/2 inch rounds
- 1 clove garlic
- The juice and zest of 1 lemon
- 2 Tablespoons olive oil
- 2 Tablespoons tahini
- Salt & Pepper

Directions:

1. Brush both sides of each eggplant slice with olive oil and season with salt and pepper.
2. Preheat the grill to 425°F using direct heat with a cast iron grate installed and close the dome for 3-5 minutes.
3. Flip the eggplant and close the dome for another 3-5 minutes.
4. Assembly:
5. Peel the eggplant skins away from the flesh and discard.
6. In a food processor, combine eggplant, tahini, parsley, garlic, lemon zest and lemon juice and puree until smooth.
7. Taste for seasoning and add salt and pepper accordingly.
8. Serve at room temperature with pita chips, pretzels, or raw vegetables.

Campfire Potato Salad

Servings: 10
Cooking Time: 10 Minutes

Ingredients:

- 2lb (1kg) new potatoes, unpeeled
- 1 green bell pepper, left whole
- 1 red bell pepper, left whole
- 1/2 red onion
- 1/4 cup mayonnaise
- 1/4 cup sour cream
- 1 tbsp Dijon mustard
- 3/4 tsp garlic, minced
- 1 tbsp kosher salt
- 1/4 tsp ground black pepper
- 1 tbsp chopped fresh dill
- 2 celery stalks, diced

Directions:

1. Preheat the grill to 425°F (218°C) using direct heat with a cast iron grate installed. Place potatoes, peppers, and onion on the grate, close the lid, and grill until beginning to soften and char, about 7 to 10 minutes, turning once or twice.

2. Remove the vegetables from the grill and let cool slightly. Cut the potatoes into quarters and dice the peppers and onion.

3. In a large bowl, combine mayonnaise, sour cream, mustard, garlic, salt, pepper, and dill. Add potatoes, peppers, onions, and celery to the mayonnaise mixture, and gently combine until the vegetables are evenly coated with the dressing. Taste and adjust the seasoning as needed. Serve warm.

Bacon Wrapped Pineapple

Servings: 6
Cooking Time: 10 Minutes

Ingredients:

- 1 cup Classic Texas Barbecue Sauce
- 1 lb bacon, cut into 4 inch strips
- 1 pineapple cut into 2 inch cubes

Directions:

1. Wrap each pineapple piece with a 4 inch strip of bacon and secure with a toothpick.
2. Grilling:
3. Preheat the grill to 425°F using direct heat with a cast iron grate installed and place on the grid. Close the dome for 8 minutes or until the bacon is crispy.
4. Brush each pineapple chunk with barbecue sauce and close the dome for another 2 minutes.
5. Serve warm with additional barbecue sauce for dipping.

Grilled Vegetable Succotash

Servings: 6

Cooking Time: 10 Minutes

Ingredients:

- 3 ears corn, shucked and cleaned
- 1 (9 ounces) package baby lima beans, thawed and rinsed
- 1 large tomato, diced
- 1 zucchini, cut lengthwise into 1/2 inch thick slices
- 1 jalapeño
- Additional olive oil for brushing
- 1/3 cup olive oil
- 1/2 tsp salt
- 1/2 tsp pepper
- 1/4 tsp cumin
- The juice of 2 limes

Directions:

1. Grilling:
2. Brush the corn and zucchini on all sides with olive oil.
3. Place the corn on a 500°F grill and lower the dome for 5 minutes.
4. Turn the corn, place the zucchini on the grill, and lower the dome for an additional 5 minutes.
5. Remove the corn, turn the zucchini and cook for 1 minute more.
6. Assembly:
7. Remove the corn from the cob and dice the cooked zucchini.
8. In a large bowl, combine dressing ingredients.
9. Add lima beans, corn, zucchini, tomato, and jalapeño to the bowl and stir to combine.
10. Serve at room temperature.

Grilled Artichokes

Servings: 4

Cooking Time: 7 Minutes

Ingredients:

- 4 large artichokes
- 2 Tablespoons olive oil
- 1 lemon
- Salt and pepper
- 1/2 cup mayonnaise
- 2 Tablespoons lemon juice
- 2 Tablespoons basil pesto
- 1/2 tsp sriracha

Directions:

1. Trim artichokes of their fibrous ends and thorny leaves.
2. Quarter the artichokes and remove the thistle in the middle.
3. Rub all cut ends with half of a lemon to prevent browning.
4. In a large steamer, cook artichokes 45 minutes or until just fork tender.
5. Brush each artichoke with olive oil and season with salt and pepper.
6. Grilling:
7. Preheat the grill to 425°F using direct heat with a cast iron grate installed and close the dome for 3 minutes.
8. Turn the artichokes and close the dome for another 2-4 minutes.
9. Serve with dipping sauce.

Arroz A La Mexicana (mexican Rice)

Servings: 8

Cooking Time: 30 Minutes

Ingredients:

- 2 small white onions, peeled and halved
- 2 poblano peppers, left whole
- 2 carrots, peeled
- 1⁄4 cup vegetable oil
- 3 garlic cloves, minced
- 2 cups uncooked white rice
- 4 cups chicken stock
- 1⁄4 cup tomato paste
- 1 1⁄2 tbsp ground cumin
- 1 bunch of fresh cilantro, chopped

Directions:

1. Preheat the grill to 400ºF (204°C) using direct heat with a cast iron grate installed and a dutch oven on the grate. Place onions, peppers, and carrots on the grate around the dutch oven, close the lid, and grill until beginning to soften and char, about 7 to 10 minutes. Remove the vegetables from the grill, chop onions and peppers, and dice carrots into small cubes.

2. In the hot dutch oven, heat oil until shimmering. Add carrots, and cook for 2 minutes, stirring occasionally. Stir in onions and garlic, and cook for 1 minute, stirring occasionally. Add rice, stock, tomato paste, and cumin. Bring to a boil, stirring once or twice. Cover the dutch oven with its lid and close the grill lid. Cook until rice is tender and liquid is absorbed, about 15 minutes.

3. Remove the dutch oven from the grill, stir peppers and cilantro into the rice, and fluff the rice with a fork. Serve immediately.

Mojito Watermelon

Servings: 8

Cooking Time: 5 Minutes

Ingredients:

- 2 slices watermelon, 1 inch thick
- 1 lime, halved
- 2 Tablespoons mint, julienned
- 1 tsp honey
- 1/2 tsp salt

Directions:

1. Grilling:
2. Place the lime halves, cut side down, on a 500°F grill for 5 minutes.
3. Assembly:
4. Cut the watermelon slices into 8 pie-shaped pieces.
5. Squeeze grilled limes over watermelon.
6. Sprinkle the watermelon with salt, drizzle with honey, and top with mint.

Grilled Sweet Potatoes

Servings: 12
Cooking Time: 20 Minutes

Ingredients:

- 5 tbsp olive oil
- 5 tbsp pure maple syrup
- 3 tbsp kosher salt
- 6 garlic cloves, minced, plus more to serve
- 2 tsp finely chopped fresh thyme leaves
- 1/4 tsp crushed red pepper flakes
- 6 large sweet potatoes, about 3lb (1.4kg) in total, peeled and cut into thick wedges
- 2 tbsp finely chopped fresh flat-leaf parsley

Directions:

1. Preheat the grill to 400°F using direct heat with a cast iron grate installed.
2. In a large bowl, whisk together oil, syrup, salt, garlic, thyme, and red pepper flakes. Add potatoes and toss to coat. Season with more salt (if desired).
3. Place wedges on the grate, being sure to shake off excess liquid, close the lid, and grill until lightly golden brown and just cooked through, about 15 to 20 minutes, turning often.
4. Transfer to a serving bowl and immediately toss with parsley and more minced garlic (if desired). Season with salt to taste.

German Potato Salad

Servings: 8
Cooking Time: 70 Minutes

Ingredients:

- 2lb (1kg) Yukon Gold potatoes, unpeeled and cut into rounds or bite-sized pieces
- 1/2lb (225g) thick-cut bacon
- 3/4 cup finely chopped yellow onion
- 1/3 cup white vinegar
- 1/4 cup sugar
- 1 tbsp Dijon mustard
- 1 tsp kosher salt
- 2 tbsp minced chives, to garnish

Directions:

1. Preheat the grill to 350ºF (177°C) using indirect heat with a cast iron grate installed and a cast iron skillet on the grate. Place potatoes on the grate around the skillet, close the lid, and roast until fork tender, about 45 minutes. Remove potatoes from the grill and set aside.
2. Add bacon to the hot skillet, close the lid, and cook until crisp, about 10 to 15 minutes. Once crisp, transfer to a plate lined with a paper towel and crumble into small pieces. Pour off the rendered fat, reserving 4 tbsp in the skillet.
3. Add onion to the skillet, close the lid, and cook until translucent and beginning to brown, about 4 to 5 minutes. Whisk in vinegar, sugar, mustard, and salt, and stir until thick and bubbly, about 2 to 3 minutes. Add the cooked potatoes, and toss to coat.
4. Remove the skillet from the grill, top with crumbled bacon, and garnish with chives. Serve warm.

Grilled Watermelon Salad

Servings: 6
Cooking Time: 6 Minutes

Ingredients:

- 4 medium cucumbers, about 1lb (450g) in total, divided
- 3lb (1.4kg) watermelon, rind removed and cut into thick slices
- 3 garlic cloves, peeled
- 1½ cups plain Greek yogurt
- ⅔ cup chopped mint, divided
- ¾ tsp kosher salt
- 2 tbsp fresh lime juice
- flaky sea salt, to serve

Directions:

1. Preheat the grill to 500°F (260°C) using direct heat with a cast iron grate installed. Peel 2 cucumbers and halve them lengthwise. Place the halved cucumbers and watermelon slices on the grate, close the lid, and grill until grill marks form, about 2 to 3 minutes per side.
2. Using a chef's knife, finely chop garlic and sprinkle with a pinch of salt. Using the flat of the blade, crush the chopped garlic, scrape into a pile, and crush again, repeating until a paste forms. Transfer to a medium bowl.
3. To make the tzatziki sauce, peel the remaining 2 cucumbers, halve lengthwise, and seed. Coarsely grate into the bowl with the garlic paste. Stir in yogurt, ⅓ cup mint, and salt.
4. Cut the watermelon into bite-sized pieces, and cut the grilled cucumber crosswise into ⅓-in (.75-cm) slices. Place cucumber and watermelon in a large bowl, toss with lime juice and the remaining ⅓ cup mint, and sprinkle with sea salt. Spoon the tzatziki sauce over top to serve.

Thanksgiving Stuffing

Servings: 8
Cooking Time: 45 Minutes

Ingredients:

- 8 ounces bulk breakfast sausage
- 4 cups cornbread, crumbled
- 4 cups sourdough bread, cut in cubes
- 1/2 cup onion, diced
- 1/2 cup celery, diced
- 1/2 cup Granny Smith apple, diced
- 4 Tablespoons butter, softened
- 2 cups chicken broth
- 1 tsp poultry seasoning

Directions:

1. Preheat the grill to 375°F using direct heat with a cast iron grate installed with the dutch oven on the grid.
2. Cook breakfast sausage in the dutch oven until brown.
3. Add onion and celery and cook until soft, about 5 minutes.
4. Add apple and cook an additional 2 minutes.
5. Stir in crumbled cornbread and sourdough bread cubes.
6. Pour chicken broth over mixture and season with poultry seasoning.
7. Dot the top of the stuffing with butter, cover, and lower the dome.
8. Cook the stuffing for 30 minutes. Serve warm.

PORK

Pork Tenderloin

Servings:4
Cooking Time: 20 Minutes

Ingredients:
- Whole pork tenderloin
- Olive oil
- Sweet & Smoky Seasoning
- Sweet & Smoky Kansas City Style Sauce

Directions:
1. Preheat the grill to 350°F using direct heat with a cast iron grate installed.
2. Trim the pork tenderloin of any excess fat and silver skin. Season with a drizzle of olive oil and a generous amount of Sweet & Smoky Seasoning.
3. Place the tenderloins on the cooking grid. Roast for 15 to 20 minutes, turning occasionally, until the tenderloins reach an internal temperature of 145°F.
4. Remove the tenderloins from the grill and place on a large piece of heavy-duty aluminum foil; wrap tightly and let rest for 10 minutes. Remove to a cutting board, slice and serve with the Sweet & Smoky Kansas City Style Barbecue Sauce.

Pork Belly & Rice Grits

Servings: 8

Cooking Time: 270 Minutes

Ingredients:

- 3 tbsp vegetable oil
- 2lb pork belly, about 1 in (2.5-cm) thick, cut into 8 pieces
- kosher salt and freshly ground black pepper
- 1 small red onion, roughly chopped
- 2 small carrots, roughly chopped
- 1 bay leaf
- 1/2 tsp coriander seeds
- 4 cups chicken stock, divided
- 1/4 cup rice flour
- 1/2 cup rice grits or hominy grits
- 1/2 cup heavy cream
- 1 cup shredded sharp Cheddar cheese or Fontina (optional)
- 1/2 cup finely chopped kimchi
- for the pickles
- 1/2 tsp sugar
- 1/4 cup unseasoned rice vinegar
- 1/2 cup thinly sliced radishes
- 1/2 red onion
- 2 scallions, thinly sliced on the bias
- to smoke
- oak, apricot, or bourbon barrel wood chunks

Directions:

1. Preheat the grill to 300°F (149°C). Once hot, add the wood chunks and install the heat deflector along with a standard grate and dutch oven. To the hot dutch oven, heat oil until shimmering. Add pork pieces, and season with salt and pepper to taste. Close the grill lid and smoke until pork has browned on all sides, about 10 to 15 minutes. Add onion, carrots, bay leaf, and coriander seeds, close the grill lid, and cook for 5 minutes more.

2. Add 2 cups chicken stock, close the grill lid, and cook until the meat is very tender, about 3 hours. Leave the lid off the dutch oven for the first hour and cover for the remaining cooking time. Transfer cooked pork to a cutting board and let cool slightly. Cut each piece in half crosswise, lightly coat with rice flour, and set aside. Discard the vegetables and reserve the braising liquid.

3. Rinse the dutch oven and return it to the grill. Open the top and bottom vents to raise the grill temperature to 350°F (177°C). Once hot, arrange the floured pork pieces on the grate around the dutch oven (not inside). Roast until the fat has rendered and pork is slightly crispy, about 15 to 20 minutes.

4. Place grits in the dutch oven and toast until just shiny, about 3 minutes. Slowly add cream and the remaining 2 cups stock in three different stages and cook until creamy and tender, about 10 to 15 minutes, stirring every 3 minutes to break up any lumps. Add cheese (if using), and season with salt and pepper to taste.

5. To make the pickles, in a large shallow bowl, whisk together sugar and vinegar until sugar dissolves. Add onions, scallions, and radishes, cover with plastic wrap, and refrigerate for 15 minutes.

6. On the stovetop in a medium saucepan, bring the reserved braising liquid to a boil. Simmer until the volume has decreased by half, about 15 to 20 minutes.

7. Transfer pork and grits to serving dishes. Stir the reduced braising liquid into the grits or as much for the desired consistency, and season with salt and pepper to taste. Serve immediately with kimchi and pickled onions, scallions, and radishes.

Pork Chops

Servings:2

Cooking Time: 70 Minutes

Ingredients:

- 4 10-oz (283 g) bone-in pork chops (about ½ in (13 mm) thick)
- 4 cups (32 oz) Sweet Tea Brine (recipe follows)
- 2 tbsp (30 ml) blended olive oil
- 1 tsp (5 ml) kosher salt
- 1 tsp (5 ml) coarsely ground black pepper
- ½ cup (4 oz) bourbon
- ¼ cup (2 oz) unsalted butter
- Apple Butter and Spiced Pumpkin Seeds (recipe follows)
- ½ cup (4 oz) unsalted butter, melted
- 8 red apples, cored
- ¼ cup (60 ml) packed light brown sugar
- 1 tsp (5 ml) ground cinnamon
- ½ tsp (3 ml) ground cloves
- ½ tsp (3 ml) ground allspice
- ½ tsp (3 ml) kosher salt
- Pinch of freshly ground black pepper
- 2 tbsp (30 ml) blended olive oil
- 1 cup (240 ml) pumpkin seeds
- ½ tsp (3 ml) gray sea salt
- ½ tsp (3 ml) curry powder
- ¼ tsp (1.5 ml) freshly ground black pepper
- 8 cups (64 oz water)
- 8 regular-size orange pekoe black tea bags
- 1 cup (240 ml) granulated sugar
- 1 cup (240 ml) kosher salt
- 1 tbsp (15 ml) black peppercorns
- ¼ tsp (1.5 ml) red pepper flakes
- 4 garlic cloves
- 4 star anise pods
- 4 bay leaves
- 2 large thyme sprigs
- 2 medium-size oranges, cut into quarters
- 1 large lemon, cut into quarters

Directions:

1. Combine the pork and Sweet Tea Brine in a large baking dish. Cover and refrigerate 8 hours or overnight.

2. Remove the pork chops from the brine; discard brine. Let the pork chops come to room temperature, about 30 minutes. Rub the pork chops with the oil, and sprinkle evenly with the salt and pepper.

3. Bring the bourbon to a simmer in a saucepan over medium heat. Cook until reduced by half, about 8 minutes. Remove from the heat and whisk in the butter. Set aside.

4. Preheat the grill to 450°F using direct heat with a cast iron grate installed.

5. Grill the pork chops until golden brown and slightly crispy on the bottom, about 6 minutes, basting occasionally with the bourbon butter. Turn the pork chops and cook until the meat begins to draw close to the bone, about 4 minutes.

6. Transfer to a wire rack; let stand 15 minutes, basting occasionally with any remaining bourbon butter. Serve with Apple Butter, Spiced Pumpkin Seeds and collard greens as a side.

7. Set the kamado grill for indirect cooking with the platesetter at 350F. Combine the melted butter and apples in a baking dish, turning to coat the apples in the butter. Bake until the apples are very tender and

the skins pop, 50 minutes to 1 hour. Sprinkle the apples with the brown sugar, cinnamon, cloves, allspice, kosher salt and pepper. Return to the kamado grill until the sugar melts, about 5 minutes. Remove from the grill, and let stand 15 minutes. Transfer the apple mixture to a blender and process until smooth. Let stand 30 minutes at room temperature or refrigerate overnight.

8.   Set the kamado grill for indirect cooking with the platesetter at 350F. Heat the oil in a cast iron skillet in the grill; add the pumpkin seeds and cook, stirring occasionally, until golden brown, about 2 minutes. Remove from the grill. Stir in the sea salt, curry powder, and pepper. Drain on a plate lined with paper towels.

9.   Bring the water just to boiling in a large saucepan. Remove from the heat and add the tea bags. Let stand 5 minutes; remove and discard the tea bags. Add the remaining ingredients, squeezing the citrus juice into the pan as you add them. Return to medium-high and bring to a simmer. Remove from heat and let stand 1 hour. Remove the solids and store in an airtight container in the refrigerator up to 5 days.

Pork Cacciatore

Servings:4
Cooking Time: 122 Minutes

Ingredients:

- 6 pounds boneless pork shoulder
- 1 1⁄4 teaspoon sea salt
- 3⁄4 teaspoon freshly ground pepper
- 2 tablespoons olive oil
- 1 large red bell pepper, sliced
- 1 large green bell pepper, sliced
- 2 yellow onions, sliced
- 3-4 cloves garlic, chopped
- 2 teaspoons dried basil
- 2 teaspoons dried parsley
- 1 teaspoon dried thyme
- 1 teaspoon red pepper flakes, optional
- 1 cup low sodium chicken broth
- 1 28 ounce can petite diced tomatoes
- 3 tablespoons tomato paste

Directions:

1. Preheat the grill to 350°F using direct heat with a cast iron grate installed.
2. Take pork shoulder out of package and wipe down with a paper towel. Season with salt and pepper.
3. Heat your dutch oven in the grill. Add in oil and let it get nice and hot. Add in pork and sear all sides for about 2 minutes; you want to create a nice sear. Add in peppers, onions and garlic. Cook for about 5 minutes stirring around using a wooden spoon.
4. Add in basil, parsley, thyme and red pepper flakes. Pour in chicken broth and diced tomatoes. Stir to incorporate all of the ingredients. Add in tomato paste and press against the pan with the back of your spoon to help incorporate into the liquid. Cover and let cook 2 hours.
5. Remove from grill. Use a large spoon and skim off the fat then go ahead and pull apart the pork or serve in large chunks with the peppers and onions. Enjoy!

Cedar Planked Pork Chops

Servings:4

Cooking Time: 18 Minutes

Ingredients:

- 4 double bone-in pork chops
- 3/4 cup canola oil
- ½ cup Lee & Perrin's Marinade for Chicken
- 1 BOU Chicken Bouillon cube
- BOU Java Rub
- Fresh bay leaves
- 2 Cedar Planks, soaked
- 2 BOU Chicken Bouillon Cubes
- ¼ cup espresso coffee, finely ground
- 2 tbsp lemon zest, finely grated
- ½ cup brown sugar

- 2 tbsp sea salt
- 1 tbsp granulated garlic
- 1½ tsp coriander, ground
- 3 tbsp chipotle chili powder
- 2 tbsp black pepper, freshly ground
- 3 tbsp smoked paprika
- 1 tsp roasted cumin, ground
- 1½ tbsp unsweetened cocoa powder
- 1 tsp dry mustard
- 1½ tbsp ancho chili powder

Directions:

1. Soak the planks for at least 2 hours in water prior to grilling.

2. Combine the salad oil, BOU Chicken Cube and Lea & Perrin's. Blend well for approximately 45 seconds.

3. Place the pork chops in a shallow pan; pour the BOU-flavored oil over the chops. Top with bay leaves. Turn the chops over to ensure they are totally coated. Marinate 3 to 4 hours; remove from the marinade and drain. Season both sides liberally with BOU Java Rub.

4. Preheat the grill to 400°F using direct heat with a cast iron grate installed. Place the soaked planks on the kamado grill for 30 seconds; flip the planks and add the seasoned chopsto the planks. Cook to the desired doneness (the internal temperature for the pork chops should reach 130 to 145°F – check temperature at 15 minutes).

5. Combine all ingredients in a blender for about 45 seconds.

6. Place into a storage container with a lid; store in a cool dry place

Potato Salad With Bacon

Servings:6

Cooking Time: 20 Minutes

Ingredients:

- 6 slices bacon, thick-cut, cooked until crisp, then coarsely crumbled
- 2 pounds red new potatoes, (golf-ball size), scrubbed and poked with a fork
- 2 tablespoons extra-virgin olive oil
- 4 green onions, including green tops, cut crosswise into thin rounds
- ¼ cup extra-virgin olive oil
- 1 tablespoon apple cider vinegar
- 1 large clove garlic, minced
- 2 tablespoons fresh parsley, minced
- 1 teaspoon kosher salt
- ½ teaspoon sugar
- 1 teaspoon freshly ground black pepper

Directions:

1. Preheat the grill to 350°F using direct heat with a cast iron grate installed.
2. In a medium bowl, toss potatoes with olive oil until well coated. Arrange potatoes around outer edges of cooking grid. Grill until tender when pierced with a knife, about 20 minutes.
3. While potatoes are grilling, put green onions and bacon in a large bowl, and make dressing. Combine olive oil, vinegar, garlic, parsley, salt, sugar and pepper in a small bowl; set aside.
4. When potatoes are tender, transfer to a cutting board and cool for 5 minutes. Cut potatoes in half and add to bacon and onions in the bowl. Stir dressing to combine and pour over potatoes. Gently toss to thoroughly combine. Serve immediately.
5. The potato salad can be made up to 2 hours prior to serving. Cover and set aside at room temperature.

Bacon-wrapped Scotch Eggs

Servings: 8

Cooking Time: 30 Minutes

Ingredients:
- 8 large eggs
- 1lb (450g) pork sausage, casings removed
- 16 bacon strips
- for the sauce
- 1 cup mayonnaise
- 1 cup coarse ground mustard
- kosher salt and freshly ground black pepper

Directions:
1. On the stovetop over high heat, bring a large pot of water to a boil. Once boiling, add eggs and boil for 4 minutes. Carefully drain, then transfer eggs to an ice bath to chill for 30 minutes. Peel and set aside.
2. To make the sauce, in a small bowl, combine mayonnaise and mustard, and season with salt and pepper to taste. Refrigerate until ready to serve.
3. Preheat the grill to 475°F (246°C) using indirect heat with a standard grate installed. Divide the sausage into 8 equal portions. Form one portion of sausage meat into a thin, flat patty and gently wrap it around one egg, making sure the egg is fully enclosed in an even layer of meat. Repeat with the remaining sausage and eggs, then wrap each egg with 2 bacon strips, completely covering the sausage with bacon.
4. Place eggs directly on the grate, close the lid, and cook until the sausage is cooked through and the bacon is crisp, about 20 minutes. Rotate the eggs a few times while cooking to ensure the bacon gets crispy.
5. Remove eggs from the grill, cut them in half, and arrange on a serving dish. Serve immediately with the sauce.

Bacon Mac & Cheese

Servings: 8

Cooking Time: 5 Minutes

Ingredients:

- 1 tablespoon olive oil
- 1 cup Panko (Japanese-style) breadcrumbs
- 12 slices flavorful smoked bacon
- 3 cups uncooked elbow macaroni
- ½ cup Cabot 2% Plain Greek-Style Yogurt or Cabot Plain Greek-Style Yogurt
- ¼ cup mayonnaise
- 8 ounces Cabot Extra Sharp Cheddar or Seriously Sharp Cheddar, grated (about 2 cups), plus more for garnish
- 2 tablespoons cider vinegar
- 1-2 teaspoons hot sauce
- 1 teaspoon Dijon mustard
- 1 medium clove garlic, coarsely chopped
- ½ teaspoon salt
- ½ teaspoon ground black pepper
- Optional extras

Directions:

1. Preheat the grill to 350°F using direct heat with a cast iron grate installed.

2. Heat oil on preheated Half Moon Cast Iron Griddle or a grill-safe pan. Add breadcrumbs and stir in pan until golden, about 1 1/2 minutes. immediately scrape into small bowl and set aside.

3. Add bacon to Half Moon Griddle and cook until crisp; transfer to paper towels to drain, then crumble or chop and set aside.

4. In large pot of boiling salted water, cook macaroni according to package directions until just tender. Drain and rinse under cold water until cool.

5. While macaroni cooks, combine yogurt and mayonnaise in blender; add cheddar, vinegar, hot sauce, mustard, garlic, salt and pepper; blend until the consistency of mayonnaise and nearly smooth, stirring and scraping down side of container as needed to help ingredients "liquefy".

6. In large bowl, toss together macaroni, cheddar dressing and bacon in large bowl, mixing well. Serve topped with additional cheese and toasted breadcrumbs. Surround with bowls of optional extras as desired.

7. Optional extras: sliced green onions, chopped Italian parsley, slivered fresh basil, raw fresh corn kernels, diced fresh tomatoes, diced bell peppers, thinly sliced romaine lettuce

Maple Bourbon Pork Chops

Servings:4

Cooking Time: 6 Minutes

Ingredients:

- 4 boneless center cut pork chops
- ¾ cup bourbon
- 3 tablespoons brown sugar
- 1 garlic clove, minced
- 1 teaspoon apple cider vinegar
- 1 tablespoons worcestershire sauce
- 2 tablespoons pure maple syrup
- ½ teaspoon ground mustard
- 1 teaspoon salt
- 1½ teaspoon pepper
- ½ teaspoon smoked paprika
- 1 tablespoon canola oil
- ¼ cup chicken stock
- 4 slices cooked bacon, crumbled

Directions:

1. In a small saucepan combine bourbon, sugar, garlic, vinegar, maple syrup, worcestershire and mustard. Bring to a boil, stirring constantly, then reduce heat to a simmer and let cook for 10-12 minutes, stirring occasionally. Remove from heat to thicken.

2. Preheat the grill to 350°F using direct heat with a cast iron grate installed.

3. Tenderize pork chops with a meat tenderizer, then coat on both sides with salt, pepper and paprika. Heat a cast iron griddle on the kamado grill and brush with canola oil and add pork chops. Sear on one side for 2 to 3 minutes; turn and cook for 2 to 3 minutes more. Slowly pour chicken stock over the chops, close bottom and top vents, and let the chops cook for about 10 minutes, until desired temperature is reached.

4. Once finished, pour glaze over top, add crumbled bacon and serve immediately.

Baby Back Ribs With Apple-bourbon Barbecue Sauce

Servings:6

Cooking Time: 180 Minutes

Ingredients:

- ¼ cup (packed) golden brown sugar
- 3 tablespoons paprika
- 2 teaspoons freshly ground black pepper
- 1 teaspoon ground cumin
- ¼ teaspoon cayenne pepper
- 3 (2 ½ pound) racks pork baby back ribs
- 2 tablespoons (about) kosher salt
- ¾ cup apple cider vinegar
- Apple-Bourbon Barbecue Sauce, warm
- 3 cups hickory wood chips, soaked in water for at least 1 hour
- 2 tablespoons unsalted butter
- 1 onion, chopped
- 2 garlic cloves, finely chopped
- 1 teaspoon paprika
- ½ teaspoon dry mustard
- ½ cup bourbon
- 1 cup apple cider vinegar
- 2 cups chicken broth
- 2 cups ketchup
- ¾ cup packed golden brown sugar
- 2 to 4 canned chipotle chilies in adobo sauce, chopped*
- 2 tablespoons Worcestershire sauce
- 1 teaspoon kosher salt
- ½ teaspoon freshly ground black pepper
- 2 Granny Smith apples, peeled, cored and finely chopped
- 1 lemon, cut in half

Directions:

1. In medium bowl, mix the brown sugar, paprika, black pepper, cumin, and cayenne pepper. Place the ribs on a large baking sheet and rub the ribs with some salt. Sprinkle the spice mixture over the ribs and massage the spices into the meat. Cover and refrigerate for at least 12 hours and up to 24 hours.

2. Preheat the grill to 300°F using direct heat with a cast iron grate installed. Sprinkle 1 cup of the drained wood chips over the coal. Place a foil pan half-filled with water on the platesetter.

3. Combine the vinegar and ¾ cup water in a spray bottle. Season the ribs with salt. Place the ribs on the cooking grate over the water-filled pan. (Don't worry if the ribs extend over the pan, as the pan will still catch the majority of the dripping juices.) Cook, with the dome closed, turning the ribs over and spraying them every 45 minutes or so with the cider mixture, adding another cup of drained wood chips at the same intervals, for about 3 hours, or until the meat is just tender. Do not add more wood chips after the 1 ½ hour point, as too much smoke will give the ribs a bitter flavor.

4. Once the ribs are tender, begin brushing them lightly with the barbecue sauce every few minutes or so, allowing the sauce to set before applying the next coat. Continue brushing the ribs with the sauce, turning occasionally, for about 30 minutes, or until the meat has shrunk from the ends of the bones. Transfer the ribs to a carving board and let rest for about 5 minutes.

5. To serve: Using a large sharp knife cut the racks into individual ribs. Transfer to a large bowl and toss with enough of the remaining warm barbecue sauce to coat. Arrange the ribs on a platter and serve with the remaining sauce on the side.

6. In a large saucepan, melt the butter over medium heat. Add the onion and sauté until tender, about 5 minutes. Add the garlic and sauté until very tender, about 3 minutes; stir in the paprika and mustard powder.

7. Stir in the bourbon then the vinegar and simmer for 3 minutes. Stir in the broth, ketchup, brown sugar, chipotle chilies, Worcestershire sauce, salt and black pepper. Add the apples and squeeze the juice from the lemon into the sauce.

8. Bring the sauce to a simmer over high heat then reduce the heat to medium-low and simmer, uncovered, until the sauce reduces and thickens slightly, stirring.

Reverse-seared Herb Crusted Bone-in Iberico Pork Loin

Servings:10

Cooking Time: 65 Minutes

Ingredients:

- 1 2.5-lb. bone-in pork loin
- 2 tbsp minced rosemary
- 2 tbsp minced oregano
- ¼ cup minced sage
- 2 tbsp minced thyme
- 6 cloves minced garlic
- 4 tbsp kosher salt
- 2 tbsp ground black pepper
- ½ cup Dijon mustard

Directions:

1. Set the kamado grill with the platesetter basket with one side indirect cooking (with the Half Moon Pizza & Baking Stone) and the other side preheat the grill to 300°F using direct heat with a cast iron grate installed.

2. Mix all ingredients for the crust in a bowl, and coat the pork loin with the crust. Place the roast on the indirect side of the kamado grill and roast for about 40 minutes. A good rule of thumb is to roast the pork for 20 minutes per pound. Once the internal temperature reaches 135°F move the pork loin to the direct side of the grill. Sear the pork for about 5 minutes per side or until the internal temperature is 145°F.

3. Let rest for 10 minutes, slice in between the bones and serve with your preferred sides.

Citrus Pork Loin

Servings: 6

Cooking Time: 35 Minutes

Ingredients:

- 11/2lb (680g) boneless pork loin roast, trimmed
- kosher salt and freshly ground black pepper
- 1 baguette, sliced
- for the brine
- 2/3 cup kosher salt
- 2/3 cup packed light brown sugar
- 4 tbsp pickling spice
- 8 cups hot water
- 1/2 cup orange juice
- for the glaze
- 1/2 cup orange juice
- 3/4 cup honey
- 3 tbsp puréed chipotle peppers in adobo sauce
- 1 tbsp Dijon mustard
- 3 tbsp ancho chili powder
- 3 tbsp canola oil
- 11/2 tsp ground coriander
- 11/2 tsp ground cumin
- 11/2 tsp Spanish paprika

Directions:

1. To make the brine, in a large bowl, whisk together salt, brown sugar, pickling spice, and water until salt and sugar have dissolved. Add ice cubes a few at a time until the liquid is no longer hot. Place pork in a large resealable bag, and add 1/2 cup orange juice and enough brine to cover. (Any extra brine can be refrigerated and saved for later use.) Squeeze out any excess air and refrigerate for 3 to 5 hours.

2. To make the glaze, in a medium saucepan, combine all the glaze ingredients. Place on the stovetop over medium heat and simmer until thick, about 10 minutes, stirring occasionally. Season with salt and pepper to taste, and set aside to cool to room temperature.

3. Preheat the grill to 350°F (177°C) using direct heat with a cast iron grate installed. Remove pork from the brine, pat dry with paper towels, and allow to come to room temperature. Season with salt and pepper to taste, then place pork on the grate, positioning it near the edge to keep the glaze from burning. Close the lid and grill until the internal temperature reaches 140°F (60°C), about15 minutes per pound (approximately 30 minutes per kilogram). Turn the meat every 3 minutes while cooking, brushing with the glaze each time.

4. Transfer pork to a serving platter and brush with more glaze. Let rest for several minutes. While pork rests, place the baguette slices on the grate and toast for 1 to 2 minutes per side. Thinly slice pork and serve with the grilled baguette slices.

Dr. Bbq's Pork Chops

Servings:4

Cooking Time: 13 Minutes

Ingredients:

- 4 boneless pork chops, about ½ inch thick
- 4 medium yellow onions, halved and sliced thin
- 2 cloves garlic, crushed
- Vegetable oil
- BBQ rub
- 4 hamburger buns

Directions:

1. Preheat the grill to 400°F using direct heat with a cast iron grate installed.

2. Add the half cast iron griddle to one side to preheat. Season the chops with the barbecue rub. Add 1 to 2 tablespoons oil to the hot griddle and then add the onions. Season the onions with barbecue rub and sprinkle the garlic powder the top.

3. Cook for about 5 minutes tossing the onions occasionally. Add the pork chops and cook 3 to 4 minutes until golden broiwn. Flip and continue tossing the onions occasionally. Cook another 3 to 4 minutes until the chops are golden brown and have reached an internal temp of 150°F.

4. Remove the chops and onions from the grill. Place a chop on each bun and top with ¼ of the onions.

Smoked Spareribs

Servings:8
Cooking Time: 300 Minutes

Ingredients:

- 2 racks spareribs, peeled
- 4 tablespoons paprika
- 4 tablespoons kosher salt
- 4 tablespoons granulated garlic
- 4 tablespoons sugar
- 2 tablespoon sugar in the raw
- 2 tablespoon chile powder
- 2 tablespoon black pepper
- 2 tablespoon onion powder
- 2 tablespoon dried oregano
- 2 tablespoon dried thyme
- ½ cup sugar
- 1 teaspoon dried oregano
- ½ teaspoon dried thyme
- 1 teaspoon granulated garlic
- 2 teaspoon kosher salt
- 1 teaspoon black pepper
- ½ cup white vinegar
- 1 cup molasses
- 1 cup Red Gold Tomato Ketchup or Mama Selita's Jalapeno Ketchup
- ¾ cup yellow mustard
- 1 teaspoon cayenne pepper
- Cherry wood chunks, for smoking, if desired

Directions:

1. Combine all of the ingredients for the rub. Evenly rub the ribs, wrap them in foil refrigerate them overnight.
2. Preheat the grill to 245°F using direct heat with a cast iron grate installed.
3. Smoke the ribs for 3 hours, wrap them in foil, return to the kamado grill and cook for another 2 hours. Remove from the kamado grill after 2 hours, and rest for 1 more.
4. Combine all of the ingredients for the BBQ sauce and bring to a simmer. Remove from the heat and base the ribs with the sauce before serving.

Pork T-bone With Walnut Bulgur Pilaf

Servings:4

Cooking Time: 25 Minutes

Ingredients:
- 1 tablespoon unsalted butter
- ½ cup finely chopped yellow onion
- ½ cup chopped California walnuts
- 1 cup bulgur
- 2 tablespoons chopped dried cranberries
- 2 cups chicken stock
- ½ teaspoon salt or salt to taste
- 1 cup apple cider vinegar
- 2 tablespoons molasses
- 2 teaspoons kosher salt or 1 teaspoon plain salt, and additional salt to taste
- 1 teaspoon crushed red pepper flakes
- 2 pork T-bone steaks, or 2 bone-in pork loin chops (about 1¼ lbs. total), about 1 inch thick
- Freshly ground pepper

Directions:
1. Preheat the grill to 350°F using direct heat with a cast iron grate installed.
2. To prepare the pilaf, melt the butter in a dutch oven (or a medium saucepan on the stove top). Add the onion and cook, stirring often, for about 3 minutes. Add the walnuts and stir about 2 minutes more. Add the bulgur and stir to combine. Add the cranberries, stock, and salt (if your stock is salted, you might not need the full amount of salt). Bring to a boil, then cover the pan and cook over low heat for 10–15 minutes, until the bulgur is tender and has absorbed the liquid. The cooked bulgur will stay warm, covered and off heat, for about 20 minutes while you continue with the pork.
3. Season the pork steaks on both sides with salt and ground pepper to taste. Grill on the grill, turning the meat and brushing it with the vinegar baste every 2 minutes. Total cooking time will be 8–10 minutes, until the meat is thoroughly cooked, with no trace of rawness in the center.
4. Serve with the pilaf.
5. To prepare the vinegar baste, in a small sauce pan combine the vinegar, molasses, salt and red pepper flakes. Bring just to a boil, stirring to dissolve the molasses. Set aside.

Cedar Plank Pork Tenderloin

Servings: 8

Cooking Time: 20 Minutes

Ingredients:

- 2 pork tenderloins
- 1 cup Basic Steak Marinade (not just for steaks!)
- 2 cedar planks (Be sure they are untreated cedar)

Directions:

1. Place the pork tenderloins and Basic Steak Marinade in a zip top bag for 30 minutes.
2. Grilling:
3. Preheat the grill to 425°F using direct heat with a cast iron grate installed.
4. Place the cedar planks directly on the grid and close the dome for 3 minutes.
5. Turn the planks and place the tenderloins directly on the heated planks.
6. Close the dome for 10 minutes.
7. Turn the tenderloins once and close the dome for another 5-10 minutes or until the internal temperature reaches 155°F.
8. Remove the tenderloins and allow them to rest for 5 minutes before slicing.

Smoked Ham On Grill

Servings:10

Cooking Time: 60 Minutes

Ingredients:

- 7-12 lb. ham, not spiral sliced
- 3 cups apple juice - water or other juice can be used
- 2 cups of apples, oranges or other fruits, cut into small pieces
- 1 cup brown sugar
- 1 tsp black pepper
- ¼ cup of bourbon
- ¼ cup of syrup
- 2 tbsp of brown mustard

Directions:

1. Preheat the grill to 275°F using direct heat with a cast iron grate installed. We recommend the apple smoking chips.
2. Fill a drip pan with the juice and fruit and place on the platesetter.
3. Score the fat portion of the ham in a checkerboard pattern, making cuts approximately 1 inch apart, and 1 inch deep.
4. Cook for approximately 1 hour for 2 lbs. of weight. During the last hour of cooking, brush ham with the glaze. Remove when the ham has reached the internal temperature of 155- 160°F.
5. Let the ham rest before serving
6. For the glaze mix all the ingredients together and let sit for 2-3 hours.

Ham Muffinini

Servings:4

Cooking Time: 7 Minutes

Ingredients:

- 4 Nature's Own 100% Whole Wheat English Muffins, split
- 8 very thin asparagus spears
- 8 slices Swiss or Gruyere cheese
- ¼ pound sliced smoked ham
- Olive oil
- Salt
- Pepper
- Dijon mustard

Directions:

1. Preheat the grill to 400°F using direct heat with a cast iron grate installed.
2. Brush asparagus spears lightly with oil; season with salt and pepper. Place on the griddle; cook 3 minutes or until lightly charred. Cool slightly; cut each spear crosswise in half.
3. Meanwhile spread mustard over muffin halves. Layer each of 4 muffin halves with 1 slice cheese. Top evenly with ham, asparagus, remaining cheese and muffin halves; press sandwiches together slightly. Brush outside of sandwiches lightly with oil.
4. Cook sandwiches on the griddle 3 to 4 minutes or until browned and cheese melts.

Cuban Pork (lechon Asado)

Servings: 8

Cooking Time: 840 Minutes

Ingredients:

- 1 (7-9 lb) pork shoulder
- 1 recipe Cuban Mojo

Directions:

1. Score the skin and fat on the pork shoulder by cutting in one direction, then the other to form cross hatches.
2. Pour Cuban Mojo over the pork shoulder, cover, and refrigerate at least four hours, preferably overnight, turning once.
3. Remove the pork from the marinade 30 minutes before cooking.
4. Grilling:
5. Preheat the grill to 225°F using direct heat with a cast iron grate installed, placing the plate setter and grid inside.
6. Place the pork shoulder on the grid and close the dome. The grill is designed to maintain this temperature for up to 18 hours.
7. After 10 hours, check the internal temperature of the pork. Remove the roast when it reads 200°F.
8. Carefully remove the pork shoulder from the grill and allow it to rest 30 minutes before slicing/pulling it apart.

Christmas Gingersnap Ham

Servings: 15

Cooking Time: 90 Minutes

Ingredients:

- 1 (8-10 pound) spiral sliced ham
- 2 cups gingersnap cookies, crushed
- 1/4 cup brown mustard

Directions:

1. Remove the ham from its wrapper, thoroughly rinse it and pat it dry.
2. Place the ham in a heat-proof roasting pan.
3. Brush the outside liberally with mustard.
4. Press the gingersnap cookies into the mustard coating.
5. Grilling:
6. Preheat the grill to 350°F using direct heat with a cast iron grate installed.
7. Place the ham inside the grill and close the dome for 1 to 1 1/2 hours.
8. Allow the ham to rest for 20 minutes before carving and serving.

Virginia Willis Pulled Pork

Servings:6
Cooking Time: 317 Minutes

Ingredients:

- 4 lbs (1.8 kg) pork butt, on the bone
- 2 tbsp (30 ml) canola oil
- 1⁄4 cup (55 g) brown sugar
- 1⁄4 cup (28 g) paprika
- 2 tbsp (30 g) coarse kosher salt
- 1 tbsp (18 g) garlic salt
- 1 tbsp (6 g) black pepper
- 1 tbsp (6 g) Piment d'Espelette or cayenne pepper
- 4 cups (.9 L) wood chips, for smoking, soaked in water
- Mama's BBQ Sauce, for serving
- 1 stick unsalted butter
- 1 sweet onion, very finely chopped
- 2 1⁄2 cups (590 ml) ketchup
- 2 cups (475 ml) apple cider vinegar
- 1⁄2 cup (120 ml) Worcestershire sauce
- 1⁄4 cup (60 ml) Dijon mustard
- 2 tbsp (24 g) firmly packed brown sugar
- Juice of 2 lemons
- 2 tbsp (12 g) freshly ground black pepper

Directions:

1. Remove the meat from the refrigerator. Combine the sugar, paprika, salt, garlic salt, black pepper and Piment d'Espelette. Rub the meat with oil and rub liberally with the spice blend. Leave at room temperature for 45 minutes.

2. Preheat the grill to 275°F using direct heat with a cast iron grate installed. Soak the chips in water for at least an hour, then wrap them in a double layer of heavy-duty aluminum foil. Place the foil- wrapped chips on the coals. (Soaked chunks are better for the long cooking time needed for full butts; soaked chips worked fine for the half butt.)

3. Place the butt in the kamado grill and cook until the internal temperature is 165°F; this should take about 5 hours. You want to keep the kamado grill temperature around 250°F; the goal is low and slow. Then, remove the hunk of meat and wrap it in a double layer of foil. Return it to the kamado grill and cook until desired doneness (for sliced pork, cook until the internal temperature reaches 180°F and for pulled pork, 190°F) This will take another 2 to 3 hours.

4. Remove the meat to a cutting board with a moat (drip groove). Cover it with foil and let it rest for about 20 to 30 minute; the temperature will continue to rise.

5. Chop the meat with a chef's knife, or shred using a pair of Meat Claws, discarding the fat and bones. The meat should fall apart and have a pink, smoky ring.

6. Place the meat in a bowl and add sauce to taste. Mix well and adjust for seasoning with salt and pepper. Enjoy, slowly!

7. Heat the butter in a medium saucepan over medium heat. Add the onions and simmer until soft and melted, 5 to 7 minutes. Add the ketchup, vinegar, Worcestershire sauce, mustard, brown sugar, lemon juice and pepper. Bring to a boil, reduce heat to simmer, and cook until flavors have smoothed and mellowed, about 10 minutes. Store in an airtight container in the refrigerator.

CPSIA information can be obtained
at www.ICGtesting.com
Printed in the USA
LVHW061528060222
710398LV00010B/232